Cardiac Surgery
in Chronic
Renal Failure

Cardiac Surgery in Chronic Renal Failure

Edited by

Mark S. Slaughter, MD

Director Cardiac Surgery Research
Advocate Christ Medical Center
Division Cardiothoracic Surgery
Oak Lawn, IL
USA

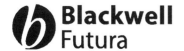

Blackwell Publishing, Inc., 350 Main Street, Malden, Massachusetts 02148-5020, USA
Blackwell Publishing Ltd, 9600 Garsington Road, Oxford OX4 2DQ, UK
Blackwell Science Asia Pty Ltd, 550 Swanston Street, Carlton, Victoria 3053, Australia

First published 2007

1   2007

ISBN-13: 978-1-4051-3132-2

Library of Congress Cataloguing-in-Publication Data

Cardiac surgery in chronic renal failure / edited by Mark S. Slaughter.
      p. ; cm.
   Includes bibliographical references and index.
   ISBN 978-1-4051-3132-2 (alk. paper)
 1. Heart – Surgery – Complications.   2. Heart – Diseases – Complications.
 3. Chronic renal failure – Complications.   I. Slaughter, Mark S.
   [DNLM: 1. Heart Diseases – Surgery.   2. Cardiac Surgical Procedures.
 3. Heart Diseases – Complications.   4. Kidney Failure, Chronic – Complications.
 WG 169 C26681 2007]

 RD598.C346 2007
 617.4′12 – dc22

                                                             2006036029

A catalogue record for this title is available from the British Library

Commissioning Editor: Steve Korn
Development Editor: Fiona Pattison
Editorial Assistant: Victoria Pitman

Set in Palatino 10/13 by TechBooks, New Delhi, India
Printed and bound in Singapore by COS Printers Pte Ltd.

For further information on Blackwell Publishing, visit our website:
www.blackwellfutura.com

Contents

Contributors

Charles A. Herzog, MD
Director, Cardiovascular Special Studies
Center
United States Renal Data System
Hennepin County Medical Center
Professor of Medicine
University of Minnesota
Minneapolis, MN
USA

Demetrios Zikos, MD
Division of Nephrology
Advocate Christ Medical Center
Oak Lawn, IL 60453
USA

Ejikeme O. Obasi, MD
Assistant Professor of Medicine
University of Illinois at Chicago
Director of the Dialysis Program
Advocate Christ Medical Center
Oak Lawn, IL 60453
USA

Kelly E. Guglielmi, MD
Division of Nephrology
Advocate Christ Medical Center
Oak Lawn, IL 60453
USA

Khalid Ashai, MD
Chief Fellow, Cardiology Division
University of Minnesota
Hennepin County Medical Center
USA

Matthew Forrester, MD
Emory Medical School
Atlanta, GA
USA

Michael A. Sobieski II, RN, CCP
Cardiac Surgery Clinical Research Center, Inc.
Advocate Christ Medical Center
4400 West 95th Street, Suite 205
Oak Lawn, Illinois 60453
USA

Rosemary F. Kelly, MD
Associate Professor of Surgery
Division of Cardiothoracic Surgery
University of Minnesota
420 Delaware Street SE, MMC 207
Minneapolis, MN 55455
USA

Rakhi Khanna, DO
Division of Nephrology
Advocate Christ Medical Center
Oak Lawn, IL 60453
USA

Sara J. Shumway, MD
Professor of Surgery
Division of Cardiovascular Surgery
University of Minnesota
420 Delaware Street SE, MMC 207
Minneapolis, MN 55455
USA

Mark S. Slaughter, MD
Director Cardiac Surgery Research
Division Cardiothoracic Surgery
Advocate Christ Medical Center
Oak Lawn, IL 60453
USA

Vidya Naidu, DO
Division of Nephrology
Advocate Christ Medical Center
Oak Lawn, IL 60453
USA

William Cohn, MD
Associate Professor of Surgery
Baylor College of Medicine
Texas Heart Institute
Houston, TX 77030
USA

Acknowledgements

I would like to offer special thanks to each of the contributing authors for taking time out of their busy schedules and sharing their time and expertise to help me complete this project; to Mr Steven Korn and Mrs Fiona Pattison from Blackwell Publishing who either called me or e-mailed me every month to check on progress, offer encouragement, and occasionally just to remind me of the project deadline; to Mrs Kathy LoBianco, in my office, who helped to compile, reformat, proofread, and tolerate each change and revision that I left on her desk; to Dr "Chip" Bolman, my mentor and friend for agreeing to review the book and writing the Foreword; and finally, to all the members of my group, especially Drs Pat Pappas, Tony Tatooles, Paul Gordon, and Mike Bresticker for covering for me and allowing me the time to complete this book. Hopefully, our efforts may result in an increased awareness of the importance and complexity of the surgical treatment of heart disease in patients with chronic renal failure.

Preface

Cardiovascular disease continues to be the leading cause of death in patients with end-stage renal disease (ESRD). The diagnosis, management, and treatment of cardiac disease in ESRD remain a difficult problem for clinicians. In 1982, Love and co-authors published "Cardiac Surgery in Patients with Chronic Renal Disease" which compiled the latest and best treatment options at that time. Amazingly, many of the clinical experiences were based on treatment outcomes of fewer than 10 patients. The chapter on valves reported on a total of 11 patients on dialysis that had a replacement over a 10-year period at the Brigham and Women's Hospital. Although important at that time, it was difficult to draw conclusions or make recommendations based on such small experiences. Clearly, we have more experience now but the morbidity and mortality of the treatment of cardiac disease remain very high in this group of patients.

Hopefully, this book will act as a catalyst to get more clinicians involved in looking for solutions to reduce the burden of cardiac disease in ESRD. Most chapters have some overlap of information. This was not an oversight but done on purpose. The book is designed to be read by a resident, fellow, or practicing clinician as individual chapters of interest. Hopefully, the information in that chapter will stimulate them to read additional sections to give them a more comprehensive review of the overall state of the surgical treatment of cardiovascular disease in ESRD.

As the number of patients with chronic renal failure and ESRD continues to expand, it is imperative that we have an increased awareness and knowledge of the effect of cardiovascular disease on their health and quality of life. It was my goal and that of my coauthors that this book will serve as a resource for some and a calling for others as we strive to improve outcomes and reduce the impact of cardiovascular disease in ESRD.

Foreword

It is my pleasure and honor to review the superb textbook entitled "Cardiac Surgery in Chronic Renal Failure", edited by Mark S. Slaughter, MD. The work focuses on an a phenomenon that is occurring with increasing frequency in the practice of cardiac surgery, namely the need to address cardiac surgical issues in patients with end-stage renal disease (ESRD). Many of our current treatment strategies are, in fact, based upon studies of a very few patients. ESRD patients have categorically been excluded from clinical trials, and, yet, data from these trials has been applied to the treatment of ESRD patients in an uncritical manner. This book is designed for the trainee or practicing physician, both for the purpose of increasing their knowledge of this complex patient group, and, hopefully, to improve the outcomes in the ESRD patients who come to cardiac surgery.

The excellent chapter by Dr. Obasi, Khanna, Nidu, Guglilimi, and Zikos provides an overview of the impact of ESRD in our society as a whole, examining the etiologies of ESRD, the natural history of this disease and the staggering morbidity and mortality rates imposed on this population by cardiovascular disease (CVD). This chapter eloquently demonstrates that this, indeed, is a unique patient population and that those practitioners venturing to care for these patients require an extensive knowledge base of the unique pathophysiology of CVD in ESRD patients. The authors point out, for instance, that aggressive screening and risk factor modification simply are not applied to the ESRD population with the same rigor as they are applied to non-ESRD patients. Much has been learned about the medical management of these patients with an eye to reducing the impact of CVD. Such factors as frequency and intensity of dialysis, treatment of anemia, blood pressure management, management of the metabolic derangements that accompany ESRD, to name a few, can potentially have an enormous impact on the mortality and morbidity caused by CVD in this population.

Drs. Herzog and Shai provide an illuminating chapter on percutaneous coronary revascularization in ESRD patients. This includes a review of the available literature in this area and elucidates some of the known differences between the ESRD and non-ESRD patient groups. The authors also examine the renal transplant population with respect to percutaneous coronary intervention and provides some excellent algorithms for management of CAD in these populations. Again, the difficult issues of the making the diagnosis of ischemia in these patients and of screening and risk factor modification are discussed. A useful discussion of percutaneous intervention in dialysis and nondialysis dependent ESRD patients, as well as renal transplant patients, is offered and can provide an excellent background for practitioners involved in this field. A plea is made for a prospective study of PCI vs. CABG surgery, in the modern era, in the ESRD population, comparing drug-eluting stents and surgical advances including arterial conduits and possibly "off-pump" CABG surgery.

Sobiski and Slaughter have written a chapter on cardiopulmonary bypass in patients with chronic renal failure. This chapter is replete with technical tips to enhance the bypass management of these patients and improve their outcomes. These pointers include factors such as limiting the crystalloid prime administered to these patients, while maintaining adequate hemodilution. The authors also advocate the routine use of intra-operative ultrafiltration for the removal of free water. Sections on electrolyte management, perfusion pressures and intraoperative dialysis complete this thorough discussion.

Drs. Forrester and Cohn added the chapter on coronary bypass grafting in ESRD patients requiring dialysis. They review the somewhat dismal literature in this area, which includes a documentation of higher mortality, stroke and mediastinitis rates in these patients undergoing CABG. Despite a higher periprocedural mortality rate associated with CABG, most studies report improved long-term survival after CABG compared to PCI in dialysis patients. The authors advocate the use of arterial conduits. They discuss the potential problem of the steal phenomenon that occurs when using an internal mammary artery ipsilateral to a functioning arteriovenous fistula. The applicability of off pump CABG (OP-CAB) is addressed.

The editor of this fine volume, Dr. Slaughter, contributes a chapter on surgical treatment of valvular heart disease in ESRD patients. A discussion of etiology is included. There is also a very helpful section on valve selection with a careful review of literature. An individualized approach is advocated, though, in general, modern tissue valves appear to be the prostheses of choice. The pathophysiology and approach to the aortic and mitral valve disease observed in these patients is well presented. Dr. Slaughter poses the question that, since most of these valve cases are not emergent, given the complexity of managing these challenging patients, might it be worth considering transferring these patients to cardiac surgery centers with (a) an interest in, and/or (b) more experience with these complex patients?

Finally, Drs. Kelly and Shumway offer a review of the surgical evaluation and treatment of uremic pericarditis. This chapter covers the incidence, etiology, diagnosis, and management of this problem, pointing out the many challenges that exist. Medical, percutaneous and surgical therapies are described, and the unique nature of uremic pericarditis and associated effusions in comparison to the non-uremic variety is well characterized.

At the outset, Dr. Slaughter states that this book is intended for the trainee and/or the practitioner in cardiology/cardiac surgery who will be caring for the patient with ESRD who has manifestations of CVD. This book will serve as an excellent reference for this field. With the increasing incidence of renal failure in our population, and the prevalence of cardiovascular disease in this population, this will constitute an ever-growing segment of the patients requiring cardiovascular care, especially at specialized centers. There is a great need for evidence-based therapies for these patients. Hopefully, this book will serve to stimulate trials of competing and complementary therapies so that the outcomes for these unfortunate patients can be improved.

Dr R. Morton Bolman, III, MD
Brigham & Women's Hospital, Boston, USA

January 2007

CHAPTER 1

Dialysis and the chronic renal failure patient

Ejikeme O. Obasi, Rakhi Khanna, Vidya Naidu, Kelly E. Guglielmi, Demetrios Zikos

Overview

The end-stage renal disease (ESRD) population has been increasing steadily in all parts of the world [1–3]. Data from the 2000 U.S. Renal Data System Annual Data Report (USRDS-ADR) show a linear rise in the incidence of ESRD, with a projected increase to more than 170,000 and a prevalence of 660,000 by the year 2010 (Figure 1). This rise has been partly due to the increasing longevity of the population contributed to by improvements in the quality of health care delivery. When the incident rate is broken down by age and the disease process, the largest increases are seen in diabetics and patients 65 years and older (Figures 2 and 3). In contrast to all other causes of ESRD, where a gradual leveling off has been observed, the incidence of ESRD due to diabetes mellitus continues to rise in a linear fashion [1]. Reasons for this phenomenon are currently unclear.

Concomitant with the rise in the incidence of ESRD has been a fall in death rates within the dialysis population. This decline has been observed in all age groups, regardless of the modality of renal replacement [1]. The declining death rate is again felt to be a consequence of improvements in health care specific to this population, including the use of kinetic modeling to quantify dialysis dose, improved anemia control with the routine use of erythropoietin and parenteral iron preparations, improved dialysis access, and use of biocompatible dialyzer membranes. Despite these improvements in the care of dialysis patients, morbidity and mortality remain unacceptably high. The five-year survival for patients more than

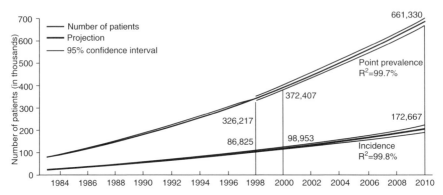

Figure 1 Number of incident and pain prevalent ESRD patients, projected to 2010. The data reported here have been supplied by the U.S. Renal Data System (USRDS). The interpretation and report of these data are the responsibility of the author(s) and in no way should be seen as an official   policy or interpretation of the U.S. Government. From U.S. Renal Data System, USRDS 2001 Annual Data Report: Atlas of End-Stage Renal Disease in the United States. National Institute of Health, National Institute of Diabetes and Digestive and Kidney Diseases, Bethesda, MD, 2001, with permission.

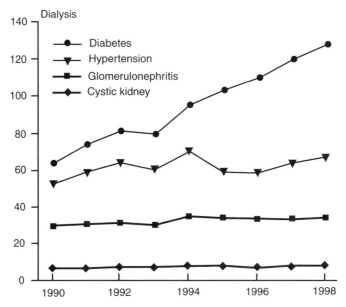

Figure 2 Incident rates by primary diagnosis per million population; unadjusted. The data reported here have been supplied by the U.S. Renal Data System (USRDS). The interpretation and report of these data are the responsibility of the author(s) and in no way should be seen as an official   policy or interpretation of the U.S. Government. From U.S. Renal Data System, USRDS 2001 Annual Data Report: Atlas of End-Stage Renal Disease in the United States. National Institute of Health, National Institute of Diabetes and Digestive and Kidney Diseases, Bethesda, MD, 2001, with permission.

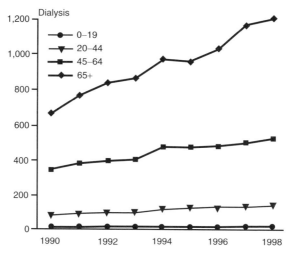

Figure 3 Incident rates by age per million population; unadjusted. The data reported here have been supplied by the U.S. Renal Data System (USRDS). The interpretation and report of these data are the responsibility of the author(s) and in no way should be seen as an official   policy or interpretation of the U.S. Government. From U.S. Renal Data System, USRDS 2001 Annual Data Report: Atlas of End-Stage Renal Disease in the United States. National Institute of Health, National Institute of Diabetes and Digestive and Kidney Diseases, Bethesda, MD, 2001, with permission.

64 years of age starting dialysis is worse than that of breast, colon, or prostate cancer [4].

Cardiovascular disease (CVD) is the most common cause of morbidity and mortality in dialysis patients, accounting for between 36 and 50% of deaths [4–9]. Even after stratification by age, gender, race, and presence of diabetes, CVD mortality is 10–20 times higher than in the general population [10]. The pathogenesis of CVD in renal failure is more complex than in the general population. Traditional risk factors associated with CVD such as old age, male gender, family history, smoking, hyperlipidemia, hypertension, and diabetes mellitus [11] are also present in chronic renal failure patients. The relationship between risk factors and CVD is often modified by confounding factors and is different, especially for ESRD patients [12,13]. There are, in addition, factors specific to ESRD and the dialysis population that contribute to increased morbidity and mortality. It is, therefore, important to evaluate risk factors for CVD in the context of chronic renal failure and recognize differences between this population and those with intact renal function.

CVD risk factors in ESRD patients

Diabetes mellitus

Diabetes mellitus is the leading cause of ESRD, representing 42% of newly diagnosed cases [4]. It is an independent cause of CVD in both the general population and those with ESRD [10]. Multiple cardiovascular risk factors such as hypertension, lipid abnormalities, proteinuria, and hyperglycemia are present in diabetics early on in the course of their illness. Many of these patients will have developed heart disease even before the renal disease progresses to ESRD [14]. There is a higher incidence of ischemic heart disease, left ventricular hypertrophy (LVH), and heart failure in diabetics on dialysis compared to nondiabetics [14]. Diabetes is associated with more severe and extensive coronary artery disease than that observed in nondiabetics [15]. These patients also have a worse prognosis after myocardial infarction [11,6], with overall mortality twice that of nondiabetics, regardless of dialysis modality [17]. CVD in diabetics is thought to be mediated in part by the formation of advanced glycation end products (AGEs), which accumulate in both diabetic and nondiabetic chronic renal failure patients [18] and are poorly removed by both hemodialysis and peritoneal dialysis [19]. AGEs cross-link and trap low-density lipoprotein (LDL) on arterial collagen [20], leading to increased vascular permeability and damage [21]. They also inactivate nitric oxide, which results in impaired coronary vasodilatation [19,21] and contributes to CVD.

Hypertension

The prevalence of hypertension in ESRD is estimated at between 60 and 100% [10]. It is both a cause of ESRD and a complication of chronic renal failure. A majority of ESRD patients have been exposed to the deleterious effects of an elevated blood pressure for several years before initiation of dialysis [10,22]. The pathogenesis of hypertension in chronic renal failure is often one or a combination of fluid retention with an expanded extracellular volume, increased vasoconstriction, or activation of the renin angiotensin system [23]. In ESRD patients, hypertension is, to a varying degree, volume sensitive. With careful attention to fluid balance and optimal ultrafiltration during dialysis, it is possible to maintain normal blood pressure in many ESRD patients [24]. Systolic hypertension is the commonest pattern of blood pressure elevation in hemodialysis patients [25], and has been identified as a risk factor for the development of LVH [26–29], which is present in 60–80% of hypertensive dialysis patients. LVH has emerged as a potent and an independent predictor of cardiovascular mortality in ESRD patients and has been associated with a threefold increase in the risk of subsequent heart failure independent of age, diabetes, and ischemic heart disease [30,31]. ESRD patients at the lower end of the blood pressure scale have also been shown to have an increased risk of cardio-vascular mortality [32,33]. This apparent paradox is explained by recognizing that hypotension is actually a surrogate marker of underlying heart failure. Heart failure is a strong predictor of mortality in ESRD patients [33].

Dyslipidemia

Abnormalities in the levels and composition of plasma lipoproteins are common in patients with renal insufficiency [34–36]. The prevalence of these abnormalities is higher than in the general population and increases with deteriorating renal function [37]. Both the prevalence and specific type of lipid abnormality vary, depending on the cause and degree of renal disease as well as the modality of renal replacement. The commonest lipid abnormality in renal failure patients is hypertriglyceridemia, often accompanied by low high-density lipoprotein (HDL) cholesterol levels. Patients with the nephrotic syndrome and those on peritoneal dialysis have elevated total and LDL cholesterol levels, with a prevalence approaching 100%. Lipoprotein analyses in renal failure patients reveal qualitative abnormalities characterized by an increase in the levels of apo-B containing LDL and very low density lipoprotein (VLDL) particles [36] even in patients with normal plasma cholesterol levels. These lipoproteins are cholesterol deficient, triglyceride rich, smaller and denser than their counterparts in patients without renal disease. This qualitative abnormality is felt to increase the atherogenic potential of chronic renal failure patients and therefore their risk of developing CVD. Levels of lipoprotein (a), another small dense lipoprotein, have similarly been found to be elevated in renal failure patients [35,38]. An elevated lipoprotein (a) level has been demonstrated to be an independent risk factor for CVD in hemodialysis patients [39].

Hyperhomocysteinemia

Plasma homocysteine levels are elevated in patients with ESRD [40], and have been independently associated with atherosclerotic heart disease and increased mortality in the dialysis population [41–43]. Lowering homocysteine levels in patients that have undergone coronary angiography with angioplasty has been shown to result in decreased restenosis rates [44], further strengthening the association between hyperhomocysteinemia and atherosclerotic heart disease.

Abnormal divalent cation metabolism

Alterations in mineral metabolism, manifesting as hyperphosphatemia, hypocalcemia, secondary hyperparathyroidism, and hypovitaminosis D are common in ESRD. Although most often viewed in the context of renal osteodystrophy, accumulating evidence suggests that these abnormalities may contribute to the increased cardiovascular mortality observed in this population [45,46]. Mitral and aortic valve calcification has been reported to be higher in dialysis patients than in appropriately matched controls [47] and correlates with the calcium phosphate (Ca_xPO_4) product [48]. The predominant cardiac lesion, however, is coronary calcification, which can be demonstrated in up to 60% of dialysis patients on autopsy [49]. Coronary calcification is more common, more severe, and occurs at an earlier age in dialysis patients [48,49–51]. The extent of coronary calcification correlates with the severity of coronary atherosclerosis [52]. Hyperparathyroidism is also felt to contribute to left ventricular hypertrophy, perhaps through cardiac fibrosis and increased cytosolic free calcium levels [53].

Anemia

Anemia in ESRD patients is predominantly a consequence of insufficient erythropoietin production [54], though it could be contributed to by iron deficiency, decreased erythrocyte survival, aluminum intoxication, and bone marrow fibrosis [55]. Untreated, anemia leads to tissue hypoxia with compensatory vasodilatation, increased cardiac output, and eccentric left ventricular hypertrophy [56,57]. LVH is seen in up to 75% of patients initiating dialysis [58], and its association with cardiovascular morbidity and mortality is well described [56,59]. An inverse correlation between hemoglobin levels and LVH by echocardiography has been noted [19,56,60], and correction of anemia leads to a partial regression of LVH [54], suggesting a direct effect of anemia. There appears to be a dose-response association between the severity of anemia, hospitalization, and mortality in ESRD patients [61–64]. Anemia aggravates preexisting coronary artery disease, with an improvement in signs and symptoms following treatment [56].

Malnutrition

Following the National Cooperative Dialysis Study in 1981 [65], malnutrition was recognized as a contributory factor to the increased morbidity and mortality of dialysis patients. Hypoalbuminemia used as a marker of poor nutritional status has emerged as a strong predictor of death in the ESRD population, regardless of dialysis modality [66–68]. It has been linked with vascular disease [69], de novo and recurrent heart failure as well as ischemic heart disease, in both peritoneal dialysis and hemodialysis patients [70]. An association between malnutrition, chronic inflammation, and atherosclerosis, dubbed the MIA syndrome, has been described [71]. The MIA syndrome has been linked with valvular calcification independent of the effect of abnormalities in calcium phosphate homeostasis [72]. That a factor other than hyperlipidemia is responsible for the accelerated atherosclerosis in malnourished ESRD patients is suggested by the concomitant finding of low, rather than high, serum cholesterol levels [13].

Inflammation

Chronic inflammation is postulated to be a cause of atherosclerosis in the ESRD population [73]. Causes of inflammation include chronic or recurrent infections, renal failure itself, and maintenance dialysis, including the use of nonbiocompatible dialyzer membranes. Inflammation is characterized by a release of cytokines, namely, interleukin (IL)-1, IL-6 and tumor necrosis factor (TNF) [74]. These cytokines mediate the increased synthesis of acute-phase proteins such as C reactive protein (CRP) and serum amyloid A protein, as well as the decreased synthesis of other proteins, such as albumin and transferrin [74]. CRP is elevated in many patients on dialysis, especially elderly patients and those with CVD [75] and is an independent predictor of mortality in these patients [76–78]. Proinflammatory cytokines, in addition to mediating a reduction in the hepatic synthesis of albumin, suppress appetite and induce catabolism, suggesting that malnutrition and hypoalbuminemia may actually be markers of an underlying chronic inflammatory state [79,80].

Other uremic factors

Left ventricular ejection fraction improves after hemodialysis but not after isolated ultrafiltration [81], suggesting a contribution of dialyzable "uremic toxins" to depressed cardiac function. Carnitine is an amino acid derivative necessary for normal beta-oxidation of fatty acids. Individuals with end-stage renal failure are felt to be at risk for carnitine deficiency particularly over time. Cardiomyopathy, muscle weakness, and rhabdomyolysis are well-described features of carnitine deficiency [82], and the finding of increased ejection fraction in ESRD patients on carnitine supplementation suggests that carnitine deficiency may play a role in uremic cardiomyopathy [83]. Beta 2 microglobulin, on the other hand, is not efficiently cleared by conventional dialysis and its accumulation is responsible for dialysis-associated amyloidosis [84]. While this typically presents as an arthropathy, it is also associated with cardiac involvement [85] and may contribute to uremic cardiomyopathy.

Asymmetric dimethyl arginine (ADMA), an endogenous competitive inhibitor of nitric oxide synthase, also accumulates in renal failure. It is recognized as a cause of endothelial dysfunction and an important risk factor for the development of cardiovascular disease in this population [86]. There are probably other as yet to be determined factors contributing to heart disease in dialysis patients, and the contribution of each of the known factors is still unclear [87].

Management of heart disease in dialysis patients

Improvements in surgical technique and in the care of critically ill patients continue to benefit ESRD patients with surgically correctible heart disease [88]. Unfortunately, CVD mortality in the ESRD population is primarily from sudden death or progressive heart failure [89], neither of which is amenable to surgical management. In contrast to CVD in the general population, classical myocardial infarction is relatively uncommon. Indeed, ischemic heart disease is less firmly associated with mortality in ESRD patients than is heart failure [90], and it appears that coronary artery disease may have its effect on mortality, mainly by contributing to cardiac pump failure [91]. Abnormal echocardiographic findings in dialysis patients, from concentric left ventricular hypertrophy to left ventricular dilatation and systolic dysfunction, are strongly predictive of the development of heart failure and death [90]. While these changes are present in many patients prior to the development of ESRD [26,92], it is possible to induce regression of LVH and systolic dysfunction if appropriate management is instituted in the first year of dialysis [93]. This in turn is associated with a reduction in the risk of developing heart failure [90]. Risk-factor modification has been shown to reduce the morbidity and mortality of CVD in the general population [94]. Patients with one or more of these traditional risk factors often have coronary artery disease (CAD) at the onset of dialysis [12]. Unfortunately, screening and treatment of risk factors are grossly underutilized in the dialysis population. According to the U.S. Renal Data System, in 1998, only 42% of dialysis patients had a lipid profile within the year [95], and 70% of polled diabetic dialysis patients did not receive glycosylated hemoglobin testing in the same year [4]. Despite the high mortality rate of dialysis patients after a myocardial infarction (reported as 72% fatality at two years of follow-up) [16], many of them are not evaluated for revascularization postinfarction and are not evaluated more frequently for the presence of lipid abnormalities [94].

Appropriate management strategies of CVD in this highly susceptible population must include aggressive screening and risk-factor modification to prevent the development of ischemic heart disease and LVH. Much of this will need to be initiated early in the predialysis period. Many of the strategies for risk-factor modification, if addressed early, have the added benefit of retarding or preventing progression of renal disease, which further reduces cardiac risk [89]. On initiation of dialysis, many patients present with evidence of underlying cardiac disease [92,96], and in these patients, the focus should shift to the stabilization of coronary lesions, regression of LVH, and prevention valvular calcification.

Dialysis patients who still smoke should be encouraged to quit, and to maintain an active lifestyle with regular exercise where possible. Diabetics should have regular glycosylated hemoglobin testing and their blood sugar control optimized as in the general population [10].

Hypercholesterolemia has been associated with an increased incidence of coronary artery disease in ESRD [97,98] in some, but not all, studies [99]. The benefits of aggressive lipid lowering in the general population are, however, well documented [37], and until a clear-cut absence of benefit is established, it seems prudent to treat lipid abnormalities in all dialysis patients. Diet therapy is of limited usefulness, as their diets are already severely restricted and patients are at risk of developing malnutrition. HMG CoA reductase inhibitors (statins) are the most effective cholesterol lowering drugs currently available and should be used preferentially in the management of lipid disorders in this population [10]. They have been shown to reduce VLDL, LDL, and intermediate density lipoprotein (IDL) cholesterol levels [100,101] by between 23 and 31%.

Effective blood pressure control is necessary for the prevention and/or reversal of LVH, and a survival benefit for good blood pressure control in dialysis patients has been demonstrated [102]. Initial efforts should concentrate on appropriate ultrafiltration during dialysis sessions, minimizing interdialytic weight gain, and keeping patients as close to their "dry weight" as possible. Drug therapy is reserved for those with elevated blood pressures despite these measures. As discussed earlier, hypotension in dialysis patients is also associated with increased mortality, raising questions about the optimal blood pressure for dialysis patients [23,25,32,103–105]. Many of these patients, however, are hypotensive because of underlying heart disease with a reduction in ejection fraction. As congestive heart failure (CHF) is strongly predictive of mortality in dialysis patients, this subgroup would be expected to have a higher mortality rate than nonhypotensive dialysis patients. Intradialytic hypotension would also increase the likelihood of acute ischemic events, contributing to increased mortality. Blood pressure management in dialysis patients should be individualized, taking into consideration patient age and anticipated lifespan, as well as the presence or absence of vascular disease [27,104]. A normal blood pressure should be the goal in young otherwise healthy dialysis patients. Angiotensin converting enzyme inhibitors are often considered drugs of choice in ESRD patients as they appear to have the greatest effect on LVH regression [106,107] and improve the outcome in high cardiac risk patients [108]. Beta blockers have also been suggested to have similar benefits in patients with heart failure or ischemic heart disease [104].

Treating anemia results in a decline in cardiac output toward normal, reduction in cardiac workload and a decrease in left ventricular mass [55,110]. This benefit is maximized with concomitant blood pressure control [111]. The fall in cardiac output is counterbalanced by an increase in total peripheral resistance that may result in hypertension [110]. A clinically significant increase in blood pressure is seen in approximately 30–40% of ESRD patients on erythropoietin [59]. Anemia correction also results in improved platelet function and, when combined with rising viscosity from increasing red cell mass, may increase the risk of thrombosis [56]. The finding of increased morbidity and mortality associated with higher hematocrit and erythropoietin use [112,113] suggests that erythropoietin use and anemia correction are not without risk. The National Kidney Foundation's [114] recommendation to maintain hematocrit levels between 33 and 36 in ESRD patients appears reasonable and should be adhered to until the risk–benefit ratio of higher hematocrits is defined.

Appropriate management of hyperphosphatemia and secondary hyperparathyroidism results in decreased risk of CAD [115]. Adequate protein intake obligates a daily phosphorus intake of 800 to 1400 mg, which cannot be removed by dialysis alone [116]. Controlling high phosphorus levels in renal failure patients depends on effective oral phosphate binder use and the suppression of excessive parathyroid hormone secretion [117]. The use of calcium-containing oral phosphate binders (calcium acetate and calcium carbonate) has been the mainstay of management for hyperphosphatemia. Their use has recently been called to question following studies demonstrating a link between high calcium loads and the development of accelerated coronary valvular and peripheral vascular calcification [49,51,118], as well as calciphylaxis [116,119]. Aluminum hydroxide is an effective phosphate binder, but its use has been limited by the potential for aluminum-induced central nervous system, hematologic, and skeletal side effects [120]. Newer polymer-based phosphate binders, such as sevelamar, are nontoxic and effective replacements to the calcium-based binders [121]. Trials are still in progress on calcimimetic agents that suppress parathyroid hormone secretion by acting on the calcium-sensing receptor [122,123].

Other less used management strategies include the lowering of homocysteine levels with the use of a combination of folic acid vitamin B6 and pyridoxine [124], replacing carnitine [83] during dialysis, and L-arginine [125] supplementation.

Recent interest has focused on "high-intensity dialysis" achieved by increasing dialysis duration, the frequency of dialysis or both [126]. Patients enrolled in these programs reported improvements in nutrition, dialysis-related symptoms, and overall quality of life [127,128]. Blood pressure control was much easier [127] with a significant decline in the need for antihypertensive therapy [129] and regression of left ventricular hypertrophy [130,131]. Phosphate control improved with some patients requiring phosphate supplementation, despite being on a high phosphate diet and off oral phosphate binders [128]. Erythropoietin requirements also declined significantly, provided patients were iron replete [128]. Finally, a region in Southern France with a large nocturnal hemodialysis program [24] has consistently reported annual mortality rates below 10%. While the number of patients enrolled in some of these programs is relatively small, the data are quite compelling and suggest that ESRD patients are inadequately dialyzed. Perhaps, high-intensity dialysis represents the most effective strategy of reducing cardiovascular risk in dialysis patients.

References

1 *U.S. Renal Data System (USRDS) 2000 Annual Data Report*. National Institutes of Health, National Institute of Diabetes Digestive and Kidney Diseases, Bethesda, MD; June 2000.

2 van Dijk Paul CW, Jager KJ, de Charro F, *et al*. Renal replacement therapy in Europe: the result of a collaborative effort by the ERA-EDTA registry and six national registries. *Nephrol Dial Transplant* 2001;**16**:1120–1129.

3 GA Posen, JR Jeffery, SS Fenton, GS Arbus. Results from the Canadian Renal Failure Registry. *Am J Kidney Dis* 1990;**15**:397–401.

4 *U.S. Renal Data System (USRDS) 1998 Annual Data Report*. National Institutes of Health, National Institute of Diabetes and Digestive and Kidney Diseases, Bethesda, MD; April 1998.

5 U.S. Renal Data System (USRDS). Causes of death in ESRD. *Am J Kidney Dis* 1999;**34**(2, suppl. 1):S87–S94.

6 *ANZ Data Registry Report 1998*. Australian Kidney Foundation, Adelaide, South Australia; 1998.

7 Locatelli F, Marcelli D, Conte F, *et al*. 1983–1992: Report on regular dialysis and transplantation in Lombardi. *Am J Kidney Dis* 1995;**25**:196–205.

8 Gomez-Farices MA, McClellan W, Soucie JM. A prospective comparison of methods for determining if cardiovascular disease is a predictor of mortality in dialysis patients. *Am J Kidney Dis* 1994;**23**:382–388.

9 Parfrey PS, Foley RN. The clinical epidemiology of cardiac disease in chronic renal failure. *J Am Soc Nephrol* 1999;**10**:1606–1615.

10 Levy AS, Beto JA, Conorado BE, *et al*. Special report, controlling the epidemic of cardiovascular disease in chronic renal disease: what do we know? What do we need to learn? Where do we go from here? *Am J Kidney Dis* 1998;**32**:853–906.

11 Kannel WB, Dawber TR, Kagan A. Factors of risk in the development of coronary artery disease: six year follow up experience. The Framingham Study. *Ann Intern Med* 1960;**55**:33–50.

12 Stack AG, Blombergen WE. Prevalence and clinical correlates of coronary artery disease among new dialysis patients in the United States: a cross sectional study. *J Am Soc Nephrol* 2001;**12**:1516–1523.

13 Lowrie EG, Lew NL. Death risk in hemodialysis patients: the predictive value of commonly measured variables and an evaluation of death rate differences between facilities. *Am J Kidney Dis* 1990;**25**:458–482.

14 Foley RN, Parfrey PS. Cardiac disease in the diabetic dialysis patient. *Nephrol Dial Transplant* 1998;**13**:1112–1113.

15 Valsania P, Sarich SW, Kowalchuk GJ. Severity of coronary artery disease in young patients with insulin dependent diabetes mellitus. *Am Heart J* 1991;**122**:695–700.

16 Herzog CA, Ma JZ, Collins AJ. Poor long term survival after acute myocardial infarction among patients on long term dialysis. *N Engl J Med* 1998;**339**:799–805.

17 U.S. Renal Data System (USRDS). Survival probabilities and causes of death. *Am J Kidney Dis* 1991;**18**:49–60.

18 Korbet SM, Makita Z, Firanek CA, *et al*. Advanced glycation end products in continuous ambulatory dialysis patients. *Am J Kidney Dis* 1993;**22**:588–591.

19 Brownlee M, Cerami A, Vlassara H. Advanced glycosylation end products in tissue and the biochemical basis of diabetic complications. *N Engl J Med* 1988;**318**:1315–1321.

20 Ateshkadi A, Johnson CA, Founds HW, *et al*. Serum advanced glycosylation end-products in patients on hemodialysis and CAPD. *Perit Dial Int* 1996;**15**:129–133.

21 Bucala R, Tracey KJ, Cerami A. Advanced glycosylation products quench nitric oxide and mediate defective endothelium-dependent vasodilation in experimental diabetes. *J Clin Invest* 1991;**87**:432–438.

22 Klag MJ, Whelton PK, Randal BL, *et al*. Blood pressure and end stage renal disease in men. *N Eng J Med* 1996;**334**:13–18.

23 Fishbane S, Natke E, Masada JK. The role of volume overload in dialysis-refractory hypertension. *Am J Kidney Dis* 1996;**28**:257–261.

24 Charra B, Calemard E, Laurent G. The importance of treatment time and blood pressure in achieving long-term survival on dialysis. *Am J Nephrol* 1996;**16**:35–44.

25 London GM. Controversy on optimal blood pressure on hemodialysis: lower is not always better. *Nephrol Dial Transplant* 2001;**16**:475–478.

26 Levin A, Thompson CR, Ethier J, *et al*. Left ventricular mass index in early renal disease. Impact of a decline in hemoglobin. *Am J Kidney Dis* 1999;**34**:125–134.

27 Foley RN, Parfrey PS, Harnett JD, *et al*. The impact of hypertension on cardiomyopathy, morbidity and mortality in end stage renal disease. *Kidney Int* 1996;**49**:1379–1385.

28 Cannella G, Paoletti E, Ravera G, *et al*. Inadequate diagnosis and therapy of arterial hypertension as causes of left ventricular hypertrophy in uremic dialysis patients. *Kidney Int* 2000;**58**:260–268.

29 Harnett JD, Kent GM, Barre PE, *et al*. Risk factors for the development of left ventricular hypertrophy in a prospectively followed cohort of dialysis patients [abstract]. *J Am Soc Nephrol* 1994;**4**:1486–1490.

30 Parfrey PS, Foley RN, Harnett JD, *et al*. The outcome and risk factors for left ventricular disorders in chronic uremia [abstract]. *Nephrol Dial Transplant* 1996;**11**:1227–1285.

31 Harnett JD, Foley RN, Kent GM, *et al*. Congestive heart failure in dialysis patients: prevalence incidence prognosis and risk factors. *Kidney Int* 1995;**47**:884–890.

32 Baigent C, Burbury K, Wheeler D. Premature cardiovascular disease in chronic renal failure. *Lancet* 2000;**356**:147–152.

33 Foley RN, Parfrey PS, Sarnak MJ. Clinical epidemiology of cardiovascular disease in chronic renal disease. *Am J Kidney Dis* 1998;(suppl. 3):S112–S119.

34 Keane WF. The role of lipids in renal disease: future challenges. *Kidney Int* 2000;**57**(suppl. 75):S27–S31.

35 Muntner P, Coresh J, Smith JC, Ekfeldt J, Klag MJ. Plasma lipids and risk of developing renal dysfunction: The Atherosclerosis Risk in Communities Study. *Kidney Int* 2000;**58**:293–301.

36 Deighan CJ, Caslake MJ, Mc Connell M, *et al*. Atherogenic lipoprotein phenotype in end-stage renal failure: origin and extent of small dense low-density lipoprotein formation. *Am J Kidney Dis* 2000;**35**:852–862.

37 Kaiske BL. Hyperlipidemia in patients with chronic renal disease. *Am J Kidney Dis* 1998;(suppl. 3):S142–S156.

38 Kronenberg F, Konig P, Neyer U, *et al*. Multicenter study of lipoprotein(a) and apolipoprotein (a) phenotypes in patients with end stage renal disease treated by hemodialysis or continuous ambulatory peritoneal dialysis. *J Am Soc Nephrol* 1995;**6**:110–120.

39 Chessman MD, Heyka RJ, Paganini EP. Lipoprotein (a) is an independent risk factor for cardiovascular disease in hemodialysis patients. *Circulation* 1992;**86**:475–482.

40 Bostom AG, Carleton BF. Hyperhomocysteinemia in chronic renal disease. *J Am Soc Nephrol* 1999;**10**:891–900.

41 Gensett JJ, McNamara JR, Salem DN. Plasma homocyst(e)ine levels in men with premature coronary artery disease. *J Am Coll Cardiol* 1990;**16**:1114–1119.

42 Bostom AG, Shemin D, Verhoef P, *et al*. Elevated fasting total homocysteine levels and cardiovascular disease outcomes in maintenance dialysis patients: a prospective study. *Arterioscler Thromb Vasc Biol* 1997;**17**:2554–2558.

43 Bostom AG, Lathrop L. Hyperhomocysteinemia in end-stage renal disease: prevalence, etiology and potential relationship to arteriosclerotic outcome. *Kidney Int* 1997;**52**:10–20.

44 Schnyder G, Roffi M, Pin R, *et al*. Decreased rate of coronary restenosis after lowering of plasma homocysteine levels. *N Engl J Med* 2001;**345**:1593–1600.

45 Block AG, Port KF. Re-evaluation of risks associated with hyperphosphatemia and hyperparathyroidism in dialysis patients: recommendations for a change in management. *Am J Kidney Dis* 2000;**35**:1226–1237.

46 Block AG, Hulbert-Shearon ET, Levin WN, *et al*. Association of serum phosphorus and calcium x phosphorus product with mortality in chronic hemodialysis patients: a national study. *Am J Kidney Dis* 1998;**31**:607–617.

47 Ribiero S, Ramos A, Brandgo A, *et al.* Cardiac valve calcification in hemodialysis patients: role of calcium phosphate metabolism. *Nephrol Dial Transplant* 1998;**12**:2037–2040.

48 Raggi P, Rienmuller R, Chertow GM, *et al.* Cardiac calcification is prevalent and severe in ESRD patients measured by electron beam CT scanning. *J Am Soc Nephrol* 2000;**11**(special issue):75A. A0405.

49 Block AG. Prevalence and clinical consequences of elevated CaxPo4 product in hemodialysis patients. *Clin Nephrol* 2000;**54**:318–324.

50 Goodman WG, Goldin J, Kuzion BD, *et al.* Coronary artery calcification in young adults with end stage renal disease who are undergoing dialysis. *N Engl J Med* 2000;**342**:1478–1483.

51 Braun J, Olendorf M, Moshage W, *et al.* Electron beam computed tomography in the evaluation of cardiac calcifications in chronic dialysis patients. *Am J Kidney Dis* 1996;**27**:394–401.

52 Sangiorgi G, Rumberger JA, Severson A, *et al.* Electron beam computed tomography coronary artery scanning: a review and guidelines for use in asymptomatic persons. *Mayo Clin Proc* 1999;**74**:243–252.

53 Lopez-Gomez JM, Verde E, Perez-Garcia R. Blood pressure, left ventricular hypertrophy and long term prognosis in hemodialysis patients. *Kidney Int* 1998;**54**:S92–S98.

54 Cotes PM, Pippard MJ, Reid CD, *et al.* Characterization of the anemia of chronic renal failure and mode of its correction by a preparation of human erythropoietin (r-HuEPO): an investigation of the pharmacokinetics of intravenous erythropoietin and its effects on erythrokinetics. *Q J Med* 1989;**70**:113–137.

55 Jeren-Strujic B, Raos V, Jeren T, *et al.* Morphologic and functional changes of left ventricle in dialyzed patients after treatment with recombinant human erythropoietin (r-HuEPO). *Angiology* 2000;**51**:1310–139.

56 Eckardt KU. Cardiovascular consequences of renal anemia and erythropoietin therapy. *Nephrol Dial Transplant* 1999;**14**:1317–1323.

57 Roger SD, Grasty MS, Baker LRI, *et al.* Effects of oxygen breathing and erythropoietin on hypoxic vasodilatation in uremic anemia. *Kidney Int* 1992;**42**:975–980.

58 Schunkert, H, Hense, HW. A heart price to pay for anaemia. *Nephrol Dial Transplant* 2001;**16**:445–448.

59 Foley RN, Parfrey PS, Harnett JD, *et al.* The impact of anemia on cardiomyopathy, morbidity, and mortality in end-stage renal disease. *Am J Kidney Dis* 1996;**28**:53–61.

60 London GM, Fabiani F, Marchais SJ, *et al.* Uremic cardiomyopathy: an inadequate left ventricular hypertrophy. *Kidney Int* 1987;**31**:973–980.

61 Madore F, Lowrie EG, Brugnara C, *et al.* Anemia in hemodialysis patients: variables affecting this outcome predictor. *J Am Soc Nephrol* 1997;**8**:1921–1929.

62 Locatelli F, Conti F, Marcelli D. The impact of hematocrit levels and erythropoietin treatment on overall and cardiovascular mortality and morbidity—the experience of the Lombardy dialysis registry. *Nephrol Dial Transplant* 1988;**13**:1642–1644.

63 Ma J, Ebben J, Xia H, *et al.* Hematocrit level and associated mortality in hemodialysis patients. *J Am Soc Nephrol* 1999;**10**:610–619.

64 Xia J, Ebben J, Ma JZ, *et al.* Hematocrit levels and hospitalization risks in hemodialysis patients. *J Am Soc Nephrol* 1999;**10**:1309–1316.

65 Lowrie EG, Laird NM, Parker TF, Sargent JA. Effect of the hemodialysis prescription on patient mortality: report from the National Cooperative Dialysis Study. *N Engl J Med* 1981;**305**:1176.

66 Acchiardo SR, Moore LW, La Tour PA. Malnutrition as the main factor in the morbidity and mortality of hemodialysis patients. *Kidney Int* 1983;(suppl. 16):199–203.

67 Owen SR, Lew NL, Yan Liu SM, Lowrie EG, Lazarus JM. The urea reduction ratio and serum albumin concentrations as predictors of mortality in patients undergoing hemodialysis. *N Engl J Med* 1993;**329**:1001–1006.

68 Spiegel DM, Breyer JA. Serum albumin: a predictor of long term outcome in peritoneal dialysis patients. *Am J Kidney Dis* 1994;**23**:283–285.

69 Malatino LS, Benedetto FA, Mallamaci F, *et al.* Smoking, blood pressure and serum albumin are major determinants of carotid atherosclerosis in dialysis patients. *J Nephrol* 1999;**12**:256–260.

70 Foley RN, Parfrey PS, Harnett JD, *et al.* Hypoalbuminemia, cardiac morbidity and mortality in end stage renal disease. *J Am Soc Nephrol* 1996;**7**:728–736.

71 Stenvinkel P, Heimburger O, Paultre F, *et al.* Strong associations between malnutrition, inflammation and atherosclerosis in chronic renal failure. *Kidney Int* 1999;**55**:1899–1911.

72 Yee Moon Wang A, Woo J, Wang M, *et al.* Association of inflammation and malnutrition with cardiac valve calcification in continuous ambulatory peritoneal dialysis patients. *J Am Soc Nephrol* 2001;**12**:1927–1936.

73 Kaysen GA. The microinflammatory state in uremia: cause and potential consequences. *J Am Soc Nephrol* 2001;**12**:1547–1557.

74 Yuen J, Levin R, Mantadilok V, *et al.* C reactive protein predicts all cause and cardiovascular mortality in hemodialysis patients. *Am J Kidney Dis* 2000;**35**:470–476.

75 Qurechi AR, Alvestrand A, Danielsson A, *et al.* Factors predicting malnutrition in hemodialysis patients: a cross-sectional study. *Kidney Int* 1998;**53**:773–782.

76 Arici M, Walls J. End stage renal disease, atherosclerosis and cardiovascular mortality: is C reactive protein the missing link? *Kidney Int* 2001;**59**:407–414.

77 Bergstrom J, Heimburger O, Lindholm B, *et al.* Elevated C-reactive protein is a strong predictor of increased mortality and low serum albumin in hemodialysis (HD) patients [abstract]. *J Am Soc Nephrol* 1995;**6**:586.

78 Yeun JY, Levine RA, Mantadilok V, *et al.* C-reactive protein predicts all cause and cardiovascular mortality in hemodialysis patients. *Am J Kidney Dis* 2000;**35**:469–476.

79 Kirchgessner TG, Uysal KT, Wiesbrock SM, *et al.* Tumor necrosis factor alpha contributes to obesity related hyperleptinemia by regulating leptin release from adipocytes. *J Clin Invest* 1997;**100**:2777–2782.

80 Moldawer LL, Copeland EM. Pro-inflammatory cytokines, nutritional support and the cachexia syndrome: interactions and therapeutic options. *Cancer* 1997;**79**:1828–1839.

81 Nixon JV, Mitchell JH, McPhaul JJ, *et al.* Effect of hemodialysis on left ventricular function, dissociation of changes in filling volume and in contractile state. *J Clin Invest* 1983;**71**:377–384.

82 Engel, AL. *Carnitine Biosynthesis, Metabolism and Function*, Frenkel RA, McGarry, eds. Academic Press, New York; 1980.

83 Van Es A, Henny FC, Kooistra MP, *et al.* Amelioration of cardiac function by L-carnitine administration in patients on haemodialysis. *Contrib Nephrol* 1992;**98**:28.

84 Fenves AZ, Emmett M, White MG, Greenway G, Michaels DB. Carpal tunnel syndrome with cystic bone lesions secondary to amyloidosis in chronic hemodialysis patients. *Am J Kidney Dis* 1986;**7**:130–134.

85 Jadoul M, Garbar C, Noel H, *et al.* Histological evidence of beta 2 microglobulin amyloidosis in hemodialysis: a prospective post mortem study. *Kidney Int* 1997;**52**:1928–1932.

86 Zoccalli C, Bode-Boger S M, Mallamaci F, *et al.* Plasma concentration of asymmetrical dimethylarginine and mortality in patients with end-stage renal disease: a prospective study. *Lancet* 2001;**358**:2113–2117.

87 Al-Ahmad A, Sarnak JM, Salem DN, *et al.* Cause and management of heart failure in patients with chronic renal disease. *Semin Nephrol* 2001;**21**:3–12.

88 Herzog CA, Ma JZ, Collins AJ. Is there improved survival of dialysis patients after coronary artery bypass surgery with internal mammary artery grafts [abstract]? *J Am Soc Nephrol* 2000;**11**:272A.

89 Jardine A, McLaughlin K. Cardiovascular complications of renal disease. *Heart* 2001;**86**:459–466.

90 Foley R, Parfrey S. Cardiovascular disease and mortality in ESRD. *J Nephrol* 1998;**11**:239–245.

91 Parfrey PS, Foley RN, Harnett JD, *et al.* Outcome and risk factors of ischemic heart disease in chronic uremia. *Kidney Int* 1996;**49**:1428–1434.

92 Silberberg JS, Barre P, Prichard S, *et al.* Impact of left ventricular hypertrophy on survival in end stage renal disease. *Kidney Int* 1989;**36**:286–290.

93 Foley RN, Parfrey PS, Kent GM, *et al.* Long term evolution of cardiomyopathy in dialysis patients. *Kidney Int* 1998;**54**:1720–1725.

94 *Morbidity and Mortality: Chartbook on Cardiovascular Lung and Blood diseases.* Department of Health and Human Services, Bethesda, MD; 1996.

95 Collins AJ, Li S, Ma JZ, *et al.* Cardiovascular disease in end stage renal disease patients. *Am J Kidney Dis* 2001;**38**(suppl. 1, 4):S26–S29.

96 Levin A, Singer J, Thompson CR, *et al.* Prevalent left ventricular hypertrophy in the predialysis population: identifying opportunities for intervention. *Am J Kidney Dis* 1996;**27**:347–354.

97 Kronenberg F, Utermann G, Dieplinger H. Lipoprotein (a) in renal disease. *Am J Kidney Dis* 1996;**27**:1–25.

98 Becker BN, Himmelfarb J, Henrich WL, *et al.* Reassessing the cardiac risk profile in chronic hemodialysis patients: a hypothesis on the role of oxidant stress and other nontraditional risk factors. *J Am Soc Nephrol* 1997;**8**:475–486.

99 Majumdar A, Wheeler DC. Lipid abnormalities in renal disease. *J R Soc Med* 2000;**93**:178–182.

100 Nishizawa Y, Shoji T, Emoto M, *et al.* Reduction of intermediate density lipoprotein by pravastatin in hemo- and peritoneal dialysis patients. *Clin Nephrol* 1995;**43**:268–277.

101 Nishikawa O, Mune M, Miyano M, *et al.* Effect of simvastatin on the lipid profile of hemodialysis patients. *Kidney Int* 1999;**71**(suppl.):S219–S221.

102 Charra B, Calemard E, Laurent G. Importance of treatment time and blood pressure control in achieving long-term survival on dialysis. *Am J Nephrol* 1996;**16**:35–44.

103 Zager PG, Nikolic J, Brown RH, *et al*. "U" curve association of blood pressure and mortality in hemodialysis patients. *Kidney Int* 1998;**54**:561–569.

104 Schomig M, Eisenhardt A, Ritz E. Controversy on optimal blood pressure on hemodialysis: normotensive blood pressure values are essential for survival. *Nephrol Dial Transplant* 2001;**16**:469–474.

105 Locatelli F, Bommer J, London GM, *et al*. Cardiovascular disease determinants in chronic renal failure: clinical approach and treatment. *Nephrol Dial Transplant* 2001;**16**:459–468.

106 Tucker B, Fabian F, Giles M, *et al*. Reduction of left ventricular mass index with blood pressure reduction in chronic renal failure. *Clin Nephrol* 1999;**52**:377–382.

107 Cannella G, Paoletti E, Delfino R, *et al*. Prolonged therapy with ACE inhibitors induces a remission of left ventricular hypertrophy of dialyzed uremic patients independently from hypotensive effects. *Am J Kidney Dis* 1997;**30**:659–664.

108 Heart Outcomes Prevention Evaluation (HOPE) Study Investigators. Effects of angiotensin-converting enzyme inhibitor, ramipril on cardiovascular events in high risk patients. *N Engl J Med* 2000;**342**:145–153.

109 Silberg J, Racine N, Barre P, *et al*. Regression of left ventricular hypertrophy in dialysis patients following correction of anemia with recombinant human erythropoietin. *Can J Cardiol* 1990;**6**:1–4.

110 Mayer G, Horl WH. Cardiovascular effects of increasing hemoglobin in chronic renal failure. *Am J Nephrol* 1996;**16**:263–267.

111 Zhender C, Zuber M, Sulzer M, *et al*. Influence of long-term amelioration of anemia and blood pressure control on left ventricular hypertrophy in hemodialyzed patients. *Nephron* 1992;**61**:21–25.

112 Iseki K, Nishime K, Uehara H, *et al*. Increased risk of cardiovascular disease with erythropoietin in chronic dialyzed patients. *Nephron* 1996;**72**:30–36.

113 Besarb A, Bolton JK, Browne JK, *et al*. The effects of normal as compared with low Hct values in patients with cardiac disease who are receiving hemodialysis and epoetin therapy. *N Engl J Med* 1998;**339**:584–590.

114 Eknoyan G, Levin N. *Clinical Practice Guidelines: Final Guideline Summaries from the Work Groups of the National Kidney Foundation-Dialysis Outcomes Quality Initiative*. National Kidney Foundation, New York; 1997.

115 Levin NW, Hulberg-Shearon TE, Strawderman RL, *et al*. Which causes of death are related to hyperphosphatemia in hemodialysis patients [abstract]. *J Am Soc Nephrol* 1998; **9**:217A.

116 Block GA, Port FK. Re-evaluation of the risks associated with hyperphosphatemia and hyperparathyroidism in dialysis patients: recommendations for a change in management. *Am J Kidney Dis* 2000;**35**:1226–1237.

117 Delmez JA, Slatapolsky E. Hyperphosphatemia: it's consequences and treatment in patients with chronic renal disease. *Am J Kidney Dis* 1992;**4**:303–317.

118 Block GA, Hulberg-Shearon TE. Association of serum phosphorus and calcium x phosphate product with mortality risk in chronic hemodialysis patients: a national study. *Am J Kidney Dis* 1998;**31**:607–617.

119 Bleyer AJ, Choi M, Igwemezie B, *et al*. A case control study of proximal calciphylaxis. *Am J Kidney Dis* 1998;**32**:376–383.

120 Alfrey AC, Hegg A, Craswell P. Metabolism and toxicity of a Aluminum in renal failure. *Am J Clin Nutr* 1980;**33**:1509.

121 Slatapolsky EA, Burke SK, Dillon MA. RenaGel, a nonabsorbed calcium and aluminum free phosphate binder, lowers serum phosphorus and parathyroid hormone. *Kidney Int* 1999;**55**:299–307.

122 Nemeth EF, Steffey ME, Hammerland LG. Calcimimetics with potent and selective activity on the parathyroid calcium receptor. *Proc Natl Acad Sci USA* 1998;**95**:4040–4045.

123 Sherrad DJ. Calcimimetics in action. *Kidney Int* 1997;**53**:510.

124 Schnyder G, Roffi M, Pin R, *et al*. Decreased rate of coronary restenosis after lowering of plasma homocysteine levels. *N Engl J Med* 2001;**345**:1593–1600.

125 Hand MF, Haynes WG, Webb DJ. Hemodialysis and L-arginine, but not D-arginine, corrects renal failure-associated endothelial dysfunction. *Kidney Int* 1998;**53**:1068–1077.

126 Chertow GM. "Wishing don't make it so"—why we need a randomized clinical trial of high-intensity hemodialysis. *J Am Soc Nephrol* 2001;**12**:2850–2853.

127 Kooistra MP, Vos J, Koomans HA, *et al*. Daily hemodialysis in the Netherlands: effects on metabolic control, hemodynamics and quality of life. *Nephrol Dial Transplant* 1889;**13**:2853–2860.

128 Pierratos A. Nocturnal home hemodialysis: an update on a five year experience. *Nephrol Dial Transplant* 1999;**14**:2835–2840.

129 Woods JD, Port FK, Orzol S, *et al*. Clinical and biochemical correlates of starting "daily hemodialysis." *Kidney Int* 1999;**55**:2457–2476.

130 Galland R, Traeger J, Delawari E, *et al*. Control of hypertension and regression of left ventricular hypertrophy by daily hemodialysis. *J Am Soc Nephrol* 1999;**10**:297A.

131 Buonocristiani U, Fagugli RM, Pinciaroli MR, *et al*. Reversal of left ventricular hypertrophy in uremic patients by treatment with daily hemodialysis. *Contrib Nephrol* 1996;**119**:152–156.

Percutaneous coronary revascularization in patients with end-stage renal disease

Charles A. Herzog, Khalid Ashai

Introduction: the burden of cardiovascular disease in patients with chronic renal failure

Patients receiving renal replacement therapy on dialysis are at extraordinarily high risk for death. The death rate for all U.S. dialysis patients in 1996–1998 was 231/1000 patient years [1]. Cardiac disease is the major cause of death in dialysis patients, accounting for about 45% of all-cause mortality [2]. Approximately 20% of cardiac deaths are attributed to acute myocardial infarction (AMI) [2]. In the United States the greatest increase in treated end-stage renal disease (ESRD) has occurred in patients with the highest risk for cardiovascular disease, older patients and those with diabetic nephropathy. There were an estimated number of 281,000 dialysis patients in 2000, with a projected number of 520,000 U.S. dialysis patients in 2010 [3]. The number of patients with nondialysis-dependent chronic renal insufficiency is considerably larger. In 1988–1994 there were an estimated number of 10.9 million U.S. patients having chronic renal insufficiency with serum creatinine > 1.5 mg/dL [4]. With this increasing burden of cardiovascular disease in dialysis patients, the number of coronary revascularization procedures in ESRD patients is certain to increase over time.

Chronic renal failure is a condition characterized by generalized vasculopathy [5]. A variety of risk factors contributing to accelerated cardiovascular morbidity and mortality in renal patients include hypertension, dyslipidemia, hyperglycemia, smoking, physical inactivity, enhanced thrombogenicity, hyperparathyroidism, and hyperhomocysteinemia. The development of left ventricular hypertrophy may be promoted by anemia and vascular noncompliance. Aortic stiffness (assessed by aortic pulse-wave velocity) is an independent predictor of cardiovascular and all-cause death in dialysis patients [6]. Premature coronary artery calcification has been detected in young dialysis patients, and the metabolic milieu of ESRD, including elevated calcium–phosphorus product may be implicated [7]. Vascular endothelial dysfunction likely contributes to the expression of atherosclerotic disease, and even a single hemodialysis run may adversely affect endothelial function [8]. In diabetic patients hyperglycemia may cause endothelial dysfunction by promoting the formation of advanced glycation end products, which may oppose nitric oxide-mediated endothelium-dependent relaxation [9]. The composition of coronary plaques in patients with ESRD may be qualitatively different, with increased media thickness and marked calcification of the affected coronary arteries compared to nonrenal patients [10,11]. The pathophysiologic significance of coronary artery calcification in ESRD patients, therefore, is not necessarily the same as in the non-ESRD population. Caution should be exercised in the application of noninvasive technologies relying on coronary artery calcification detection as a surrogate for coronary artery disease in ESRD patients, although one recent small retrospective study suggests a potential role for electron beam computerized tomography in these patients [12].

It is difficult to accurately apportion the absolute percentage of morbidity and mortality in ESRD patients directly attributable to "obstructive" coronary artery disease. Although this distinction may strike some as overly pedantic, it does have implications for the potential magnitude of therapeutic benefit derived from coronary revascularization. The largest cause of cardiac death identified in the U.S. Renal Data System (USRDS) database is "cardiac arrest, cause unknown," which accounted for 47% of all cardiac deaths in U.S. dialysis patients from 1996 to 1998 [2]. The presence of left ventricular hypertrophy and the concomitant occurrence of abnormalities in myocardial ultrastructure and function, including interstitial fibrosis, decreased perfusion reserve, and diminished ischemia tolerance, [13–16] may make ESRD patients particularly vulnerable to sudden cardiac death. The nonphysiologic nature of conventional hemodialysis schedules (usually administered thrice weekly in the United States on Monday, Wednesday, Friday or Tuesday, Thursday, Saturday) may also contribute to increased cardiac death, based on Bleyer *et al.*'s finding that significantly higher cardiac mortality occurs on Mondays (and, to a lesser extent, on the other dialysis day after the long interdialytic weekend, Tuesday) [17]. It is unclear when these excess deaths temporally occur in relation to the scheduled hemodialysis run. It is tempting to implicate the nonphysiologic effects of rapid volume and electrolyte shifts, but these can only be partly to blame, as the cardiac death rate (158 deaths per 1000 patient years) of diabetic patients receiving peritoneal dialysis (without the attendant rapid volume changes) is actually higher than for diabetic hemodialysis patients (126 deaths per 1000 patient years) [2]. Preliminary data indicate worse long-term survival after AMI for patients receiving peritoneal versus hemodialysis. In a comorbidity-adjusted Cox model, the risk of all-cause death after AMI was 19% lower for hemodialysis versus peritoneal dialysis [18]. It is plausible, but unproven, that long-duration quotidian hemodialysis may yield improved survival in ESRD patients; the favorable Tassin (France) experience with long-duration dialysis offers one scenario for improved cardiovascular outcomes in ESRD patients.

AMI in dialysis patients is a catastrophic clinical event associated with dismal long-term survival [19–23]. Based on USRDS data, we reported a 1-year mortality of 59% and 73% 2-year mortality for 34,189 dialysis patients in the United States sustaining AMI in 1977 to 1995 [19]. Figure 1 graphically displays the poor long-term outcome of dialysis patients after AMI. Even more striking was the poor survival of patients treated in the "era of reperfusion": the 1- and 2-year mortality of patients with AMI in 1990–1995 were, respectively, 62% and 74% [19]. The poor outcome of dialysis patients sustaining AMI may, in part, reflect inadequate treatment, including underutilization of intravenous thrombolytic therapy [24,25] and beta blockers [22,25]. The unfortunate exclusion of ESRD patients from past clinical trials on the treatment of acute coronary syndromes may have abetted a nihilistic approach to the treatment of dialysis patients, as data on the safety and efficacy of modern pharmacologic agents (which have been shown to benefit nonrenal patients) for the treatment of acute coronary syndromes are nonexistent in dialysis patients.

We have examined the temporal pattern of AMI occurrence in relation to initiation of renal replacement therapy. Figure 2 shows the cumulative

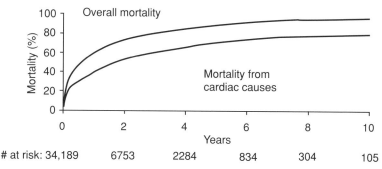

Figure 1 Estimated mortality of dialysis patients after acute myocardial infarction. (From reference [19].)

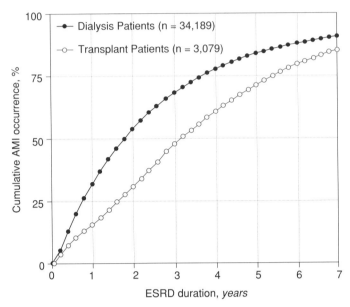

Figure 2 Cumulative occurrence of acute myocardial infraction related to duration of end-stage renal disease. (From reference [23], with permission.)

occurrence of AMI in a cohort of 34,189 dialysis patients and 3079 renal transplant recipients hospitalized for AMI in the United States. There appears to be an early hazard of AMI related to dialysis initiation, as 52% of infarcts occurred within 2 years of dialysis initiation (vs 29% in transplant recipients). Dialysis may be a "stress test" for occult coronary artery disease or it conceivably may promote the development of acute coronary syndromes. This temporal clustering has implications for the diagnosis and treatment of ischemic heart disease in dialysis patients. In the United States "high cardiac risk" renal transplant candidates are typically screened for occult coronary artery disease. By the same logic, the highest risk ESRD group for cardiac disease, newly dialyzed patients, should also be evaluated (irrespective of transplant candidacy). It may be possible to identify a subset of dialysis patients at the highest risk for death, perhaps with outpatient testing for the presence of increased serum cardiac troponin I and troponin T, as both appear to prospectively identify dialysis patients at increased risk for mortality [26,27].

   The detection and treatment of coronary artery disease before renal transplantation can potentially reduce the risk of adverse cardiac events. Current guidelines of the American Society of Transplantation recommend that patients at high risk for ischemic heart disease be screened before renal transplantation [28,29]. Figure 3 summarizes the algorithm employed at our own medical center for the evaluation and treatment of ischemic

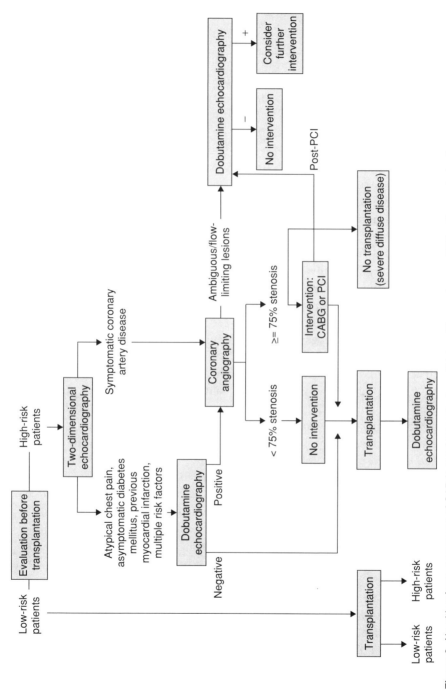

Figure 3 Algorithm for management of CAD in renal transplant candidates. (From reference [30], with permission.)

heart disease in renal transplant candidates. In our institution, we rely on dobutamine stress echocardiography for the noninvasive evaluation of ESRD patients, because of older published data regarding the poor sensitivity of pharmacologic stress nuclear imaging for the prediction of angiographically defined "clinically significant" coronary artery disease, and data from our own prospective study on dobutamine stress echocardiography and quantitative coronary angiography in renal transplant candidates [31–33]. Under the best of circumstances, all noninvasive imaging modalities (including dobutamine stress echocardiography) are imperfect in ESRD patients, and local expertise should determine the individual institutional approach. We are currently completing a study on the concordance of pharmacologic stress nuclear and echocardiographic imaging in ESRD patients; preliminary data suggest lower sensitivity of stress nuclear imaging for detection of coronary artery disease [34]. If the primary goal of screening ESRD patients before transplantation is solely risk stratification, and not prediction of "significant" obstructive coronary artery disease at angiography, published data support the use of stress nuclear or echocardiographic imaging. Unfortunately, this superficially trivial distinction presents a thorny management issue in ESRD patients, particularly if the restenosis rate after successful percutaneous coronary intervention (PCI) is high, and repeat noninvasive imaging is relied on for the subsequent detection of restenosis.

The optimal treatment of ischemic heart disease in ESRD patients before renal transplantation is controversial, because there are no published prospective clinical trials comparing "modern" (i.e., effective) medical therapy to surgical or percutaneous coronary revascularization in ESRD patients. The closest approximation to such a study was published by Manske *et al.* [35], comparing the outcome of 26 angina-free diabetic renal transplant candidates (with preserved left ventricular systolic performance, no left main disease, and at least one coronary artery stenosis in the proximal two-thirds of the vessel with a visually estimated stenosis of >75% *and* a translesional pressure gradient of 15 mm Hg) randomized to either medical therapy with nifedipine and aspirin or "prophylactic" coronary revascularization with PTCA (if judged technically feasible) or coronary artery bypass surgery (CAB). Ten of 13 medically treated versus two (both PTCA) of 13 revascularized patients had a prespecified cardiac endpoint (unstable angina, MI, or cardiac death) at a median time of 8.4 months after randomization ($p = 0.002$), and the trial was prematurely terminated. In retrospect, the medical treatment arm employed questionable therapy, given the benefits associated with beta-blocker therapy in ischemic heart disease. The revascularization arm of the study treated the eight PTCA and five CAB patients as having received equivalent therapies, a problematic assumption for a population of ESRD patients. Interestingly, noninvasive evaluation played no role in this clinical trial.

The accurate interpretation of studies on procedural outcome in dialysis patients is a potentially treacherous problem if nonfatal endpoints commonly employed in nonrenal patients are used in survival analyses. In the nonrenal population, the risk of all-cause death in the first year after percutaneous coronary revascularization is low compared to the risk of restenosis, making a comparison of restenosis risk a reasonable primary endpoint for a trial of PTCA and coronary stents. If a large number of patients die, however, in the first 6 months, repeat revascularization would be a meaningless endpoint, since the "best" outcome (i.e., lowest repeat revascularization rate) could occur in the group with the highest death rate. We compared the repeat revascularization and death rates in 8724 dialysis patients receiving CAB, 5470 PTCA alone, and 7118 with coronary stents in the United States from 1995 to 1999 [36]. Only 21% of patients receiving stents underwent repeat coronary revascularization of any type (CAB, PTCA, or stent) with a repeat revascularization rate of 218/1000 patient years. The death rate, however, was 360/1000 patient years (and in the ESRD population, all-cause mortality mirrors cardiac mortality). Figures 4a,b demonstrate the importance of using a composite endpoint (including death) in the evaluation of procedural outcome.

The clinical follow-up of dialysis patients (including those on the transplant wait list) after PCI presents special problems. One major conundrum is determining the cause of recurrent angina or dyspnea in a dialysis patient following an initially successful procedure. Dialysis patients, with their high prevalence of left ventricular hypertrophy ($\geq 75\%$) and attendant abnormalities of diastolic function, are sensitive to changes in left ventricular preload. The average American hemodialysis patient is exposed to one day of increased volume stress after the long interdialytic weekend. The accurate determination of the etiology of anginal symptoms in a dialysis patient by subjective criteria is practically impossible—volume overload and obstructive coronary artery disease (including restenosis after PTCA or stent) can produce identical symptoms: *angina or dyspnea*. If eating a pepperoni pizza on a Sunday night and in-stent restenosis produce the same symptoms (angina/dyspnea), it is plausible that a clinician might choose the wrong therapy when confronted by a dialysis patient with anginal symptoms. For this reason, in dialysis patients undergoing PCI, the subsequent occurrence of anginal symptoms cannot be used as a reliable surrogate for restenosis. Our own data on repeat coronary revascularization and competing death risk [36] after coronary intervention are also nettlesome,

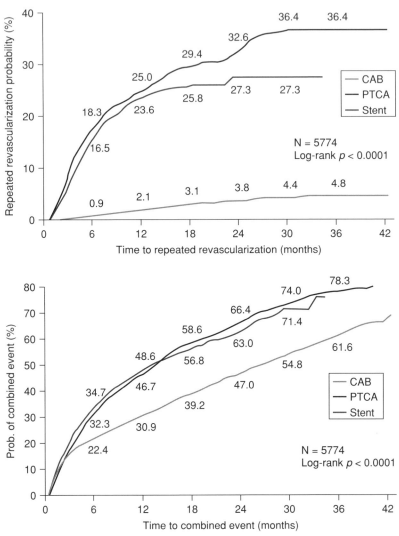

Figure 4 (a) Probability of repeat coronary revascularization after an index coronary revascularization procedure in dialysis patients with diabetic ESRD. (b) Probability of repeat coronary revascularization or death after an index coronary revascularization procedure in dialysis patients with diabetic ESRD. (From reference [37].)

as the question is raised of how many deaths were actually due to "occult" restenosis. Recurrent episodes of myocardial ischemia may be either "silent," or equally probable, its clinical recognition obfuscated by volume status (including the effects of illicit pepperoni pizza, Virginia ham, and the like). For this reason, in our own program at Hennepin County Medical Center, *all* dialysis patients undergoing PCIs with PTCA or stents have dobutamine stress echocardiography performed at time intervals chosen to detect occult restenosis (usually 12 to 16 weeks postprocedure).

ESRD patients awaiting cadaveric renal transplants after successful PCI pose an additional problem: progression of coronary artery disease (apart from restenosis) while on the transplant wait list, a time period which can easily span 3 years. In our own center, we arbitrarily reevaluate our "high cardiac risk" wait list patients at 12–18 month intervals. Obviously, renal transplantation does not cure coronary artery disease, and similar issues regarding routine "surveillance" noninvasive stress imaging in renal transplant recipients are currently unresolved. In all ESRD patients (transplant and dialysis), aggressive attempts at prevention of coronary artery disease are appropriate [38]. In some instances, we have begun to reevaluate our asymptomatic diabetic renal transplant recipients 3–5 years posttransplant. Although cardiac disease is the largest identified cause of death in renal transplant recipients, their absolute death rate (29/1000 patient years for all nondiabetic patients with functioning transplants in1996–1998, and 58/1000 patient years in diabetic patients) [1] is considerably lower than dialysis patients.

PCI in dialysis patients

Challenges

Patients with chronic renal failure are a challenging group for coronary intervention. Although the increased risk of PCI in these patients is partly explainable by increased comorbidity and unfavorable lesion types [39], there is still an increased risk of death attributable to ESRD. In comparison to the non-ESRD population, there are *no* "low-risk" ESRD patients undergoing PCI. Conceptually, these patients should be viewed in the context of published clinical trial data in "high-risk" PCI patient subsets. Unfortunately, ESRD patients have been excluded from large-scale clinical trials, including studies of PCI and adjunctive pharmacologic agents. Generally, the highest risk patient groups derive the most potential benefit (and probably suffer the highest complication rate) from effective therapies. As a group at particularly high risk for cardiovascular morbidity and mortality, ESRD patients should be an ideal patient population for clinical trials of promising therapies, provided our frame of reference is not "conventional low-risk" PCI.

Outcomes

Since no large-scale prospective randomized trials are available, data concerning the outcomes of PCI in patients with ESRD are limited to retrospective analyses of relatively small numbers of patients treated in single centers or identified from large databases. Typically, the results of PCI in ESRD patients have been compared to results after CAB or compared to PCI in patients with normal renal function in a retrospective case control design. Outcome analysis is based on mortality and cardiovascular events (frequently including a composite of all-cause or cardiac death, MI and repeat target vessel revascularization, also known as MACE or major adverse cardiac events) both in-hospital and posthospital discharge. Table 1 summarizes outcome data presented in the accompanying text.

Simsir *et al.* [44] compared 22 consecutive ESRD patients undergoing CAB and 19 patients undergoing PTCA. LIMA grafting was used in 16 of 22 patients. CAB patients had longer in-hospital stay and longer ICU stay. In-hospital mortality rate was comparable (4.5% in CAB vs 5.3% in PTCA group). Survival at 18 months was comparable ($67 \pm 17\%$ in CAB vs $69 \pm 14\%$ in PTCA group), but patients undergoing CAB had better cardiac event-free survival at 18 months (87% vs 40%).

Koyanagi *et al.* [45] compared the long-term outcome of 23 dialysis patients undergoing CAB (91% received LIMA grafts) to 20 dialysis patients undergoing PTCA 1984–1992. The 5-year event-free survival for the combined endpoints of cardiac death, repeat coronary revascularization, or AMI was 70% for the CAB group versus 18% after PTCA ($p < 0.001$).

Takeshita *et al.* [47] performed PTCA on 21 lesions in 15 ESRD patients with procedural success in 76% in the "present" era. The restenosis rate was 6 of 16 lesions studied (38%), not statistically different from nonuratemic patients (32%). The restenosis rate was higher in patients on dialysis for a longer duration.

Schoebel *et al.* [55] assessed restenosis in 20 ESRD patients receiving PTCA compared to case-matched controls without renal disease. This is the *only* study where restenosis was assessed clinically as well as angiographically in *all* patients postangioplasty, regardless of symptoms. ESRD patients had a higher restenosis rate (60% vs 35%), but this was not statistically significant (reflecting the small sample size). Of note, they also had a higher plasma fibrinogen, and smaller reference vessel diameter.

Le Feuvre *et al.* [41] performed a case control study of 100 ESRD patients and 100 control patients with normal renal function undergoing PCI. Coronary stents were used on average in 40% of patients. PCI was successful in 90% of ESRD patients and 93% of controls. Cardiac death was higher in ESRD patients in the follow-up period at 1 year (11% vs 2%). The restenosis rate was comparable (31% vs 28%), although only symptomatic patients were catheterized. There was a statistically insignificant increase in the composite endpoint of cardiac death, MI and revascularization in the ESRD group. All patients received ASA, heparin, and ticlopidine, and 5%

Table 1 Coronary revascularization in dialysis patients.

	Dialysis Pts (n = PCI if not specified)	Type of study	Periprocedural success	Results	Comment
Asinger [39]	77	Case control retrospective	89%	33% 2 yr mortality; 46% 2 yr MACE	No diff. in ESRD vs CRF
Agirbasli [40]	122 PCI 130 CAB	Retrospective analysis	99%	PCI: 23% 1 yr mortality; 51% 1 yr MACE; 11% stent use;1 yr f/u	1 yr CAB mortality: 27% 1 yr PCI mortality: 23%
Le Feuvre [41]	100	Case control retrospective	91%	11% 1 yr mortality; 42% 1 yr MACE; 40% stent use; 1 yr f/u	Ticlopidine use, dialysis vs nondialysis, stent vs nonstent
Azar [42]	34	Case control retrospective	91%	18% 9 mo mortality; 9 mo f/u; 35% TVR at 9 mo	
Ohmoto [43]	92 PCI 42 CAB	Retrospective	87%	1% in-hospital death (PCI and 15% (CAB); 59% restenosis post-PCI; 5yr survival 57% after PCI vs 62% after CAB	
Simsir [44]	19 PTCA 22 CAB	Retrospective		67% survival post-CAB and 69% post-CAB at 18 mo; cardiac event-free survival 87% after CAB and 40% PTCA	
Koyanagi [45]	20 PTCA 23 CAB	Retrospective analysis	76%	PTCA: 18% 5 yr cardiac event-free survival; 70% after CAB	70% restenosis in PTCA group
Rinehart [46]	24 PTCA 60 CAB	Retrospective	92%	51% 2 yr survival after PTCA; 66% 2 yr survival after CAB	69% restenosis rate (9/13 restudied)

(Continued)

Table 1 (*Continued*)

	Dialysis Pts (n = PCI if not specified)	Type of study	Periprocedural success	Results	Comment
Takeshita [47]	15	Retrospective	78%	38% restenosis	
Kahn [48]	17	Retrospective	96%	20% in-hospital complication with 11% in-hospital death	Restenosis in 81% (26 of 32) vessels dilated
Rubenstein [49]	27	Case control retrospective	89.5%	27% 1 yr mortality; 51% 1 yr MACE	Stent use 31%; 15% restenosis; no difference in dialysis and nondialysis patients
Szczech [50]	163 PCI 244 CAB	Retrospective analysis (New York state clinical databases)		PTCA survival: 1 yr 76%, 2 yr 52%, 3 yr 46% CAB survival: 1 yr 82%, 2 yr 75%, 3 yr 62%	PCI group mostly PTCA (no. of stents not given) PCI vs CAB: dialysis and CRF groups
Ahmed [51]	21	Retrospective	57%	33% 1 yr mortality	14% in-hospital mortality and 19% in-hospital nonfatal MI
Herzog (1999) [52]	6887 PTCA 7419 CAB	Retrospective (USRDS database)		PTCA: 2 yr 53% survival CAB: 2 yr 57% survival	PTCA vs CAB (9% decreased death risk for CAB)

First author [ref]	N	Study type		Results	Comments
Herzog (2001) [53]	5470 PTCA 7118 STENT 8724 CAB	Retrospective (USRDS database)		PTCA: 2 yr 49% survival STENT: 2 yr 51% survival CAB(IMG−): 2 yr 50% survival CAB(IMG+): 2 yr 60% survival	STENT vs PTCA 9% decreased death risk; CAB (IMG−) vs PTCA 10% decreased death risk; CAB (IMG+) vs PTCA 25% decreased death risk
Marso [54]	23	Retrospective case control		3 yr 61% mortality (vs 11% controls); TVR 41% at 6 mo (vs 11% controls)	
Schoebel [55]	20	Case control		60% restenosis rate after PTCA vs 35% in controls	All dialysis patients had angiography after PTCA
Gruberg [56]	95	Retrospective	"92%" (non-Q-wave MI excluded)	49% 1 yr mortality 59% 1 yr MACE	High rate of periprocedural non-Q-wave MI (17.6%)
Best [57]	50	Retrospective	92%	24% 1 yr mortality 39% 1 yr MACE	Stent use 68%; severity of renal failure predictive of outcome

CAB, coronary artery bypass; CRF, chronic renal failure; ESRD, end-stage renal disease; IMG, internal mammary graft; MACE, major adverse cardiac events; PCI, percutaneous coronary interventions; PCTA, percutaneous transluminal coronary angioplasty.

of ESRD patients received abciximab. The ESRD study population was unusual, as only 23% of patients had diabetes. There were no data pertaining to all-cause death. In a prior publication Le Feuvre *et al.* [58] identified from their database 27 dialysis patients receiving stents, 250 nondialysis stent patients, 60 dialysis patients with PTCA alone, and 864 nondialysis patients with PTCA alone. At 1-year follow-up, cardiac death occurred in 15% of the dialysis patients with stents and 12% of dialysis patients following successful PTCA. In the nondialysis PCI groups, cardiac death occurred in 1.6% of the stent patients ($p < 0.002$ vs dialysis) and 4% of the PTCA group. There were no data pertaining to all-cause death.

Asinger *et al.* [39] studied 77 patients with CRF (49 ESRD and 28 patients with CRF not on dialysis) and matched them to nonrenal controls. CRF patients had more complex, "unfavorable" lesions (i.e., B2 and C). Procedural success was slightly lower in the CRF group (89% vs 97%). There was no difference in the restenosis rate, target vessel revascularization (TVR), or target lesion revascularization (TLR). The 2-year cardiac event-free survival was lower in the CRF group (54% vs 69%). The risk of competing death, however, was high in the ESRD group (39% of patients died in the follow-up vs only 4% in the control group).

Agirbasli *et al.* [40] retrospectively reviewed outcomes in 252 ESRD patients at Emory undergoing PCI or CAB. PTCA was performed in 122 patients (151 lesions). There were fewer in-hospital deaths in the PTCA group (1.6% vs 6.9%). Although 1-year mortality was similar in two groups (23% in PTCA group vs 27% in CAB), PTCA group had more myocardial infarctions at 1 year (4.7% vs 2.9%) and more need for PTCA (16% vs 2.1%) or CAB (7.5% vs 0%).

Azar *et al.* [42], in a well-designed retrospective study, compared the outcome of 34 dialysis patients receiving coronary stents in 40 lesions to nonrenal control patients with 80 lesions matched for treatment site, diabetic status, lesion length, and reference vessel diameter. ASA, ticlopidine, and heparin were used in most patients. Angiographic success was achieved in 91% of ESRD patients and 97% of controls. In-hospital death was higher in the ESRD group (5.9% vs 1.3%). At 9-month follow-up, TLR was 35% in the ESRD (and 18% mortality) versus 16% in the controls (and 2% mortality).

Ahmed *et al.* [51] analyzed outcomes of 21 ESRD patients treated with angioplasty. Procedural success was achieved in only 57% (12 of 21) in the prestent era. Three out of these 21 patients (14%) died and four (19%) had nonfatal MI in the hospital. At 1 year, four more patients had died with a total 1-year mortality of 33%, and 60% of survivors had recurrent angina. In the 15 patients who were discharged with patent vessels postPTCA, four (27%) died of cardiac deaths (three sudden and one MI).

Reusser *et al.* [59] matched a retrospective cohort of 13 dialysis patients undergoing PTCA to 13 controls. At 2 years, 50% of the dialysis group experienced a cardiac event (angina recurrence, MI, cardiac death, or CAB) versus 15% of the controls.

Kahn *et al.*'s [48] paper is of historical interest, as it was the first widely read publication to highlight unfavorable PCI outcomes in dialysis patients (the first publication was probably Kober *et al.* published in German [60]). They reported a series of 17 chronic dialysis patients with 47 of 49 vessels successfully dilated. The in-hospital mortality was 11.7%, and at 20-month follow-up the mortality was 53%. In the 15 patients discharged alive during a mean follow-up of 20 months seven more patients died with total mortality of 53%. Of the 15 patients discharged alive after PTCA, angina recurred in 12 of 15 patients. In 26 of 32 (81%) dilated vessels, restenosis was demonstrated angiographically.

Ohmoto [43] reported the outcome of 92 dialysis patients receiving PTCA and 47 undergoing CAB surgery in a retrospective series of patients treated in 1983–1997. PTCA alone was used in 76% of patients (with stents in 17%). PCI was initially successful in 87% of patients. Restenosis was present in 40 of 68 (59%) patients having repeat angiography, and the authors implied that routine angiography was performed at 3–6 months post-PCI (but it is unclear what happened to the other PCI patients in the first 6 months of follow-up). The in-hospital death for PTCA was 1% for PTCA versus 15% for CAB. The long-term survival, however, was similar to 5-year 57% survival after PCI and 62% after CAB (and considerably better than other reported series). Compete revascularization (by either method) was associated with better outcome. On long-term follow-up, in the PCI group 39 patients had a second PTCA and 19 underwent CAB (38-month follow-up), and 12 patients had PTCA and 3 repeat CAB in the CAB group (51-month follow-up).

Rinehart *et al.* [46] studied 84 ESRD (without prior revascularization), 24 of whom underwent PTCA. Only 7 of the 60 CAB patients received LIMA grafts. The PTCA procedural success was 92%. The 2-year survival was 51% in the PTCA group and 66% after CAB, but this was not statistically significant. At 6-month follow-up, 60% of the PTCA group and 23% of the CAB patients had experienced a cardiac event (recurrent angina, MI, or cardiac death). At 66 months only 12% of the PTCA group had not experienced a cardiac event versus 53% of the CAB group. Only 13 out of 24 PTCA patients were restudied and 9 of these had evidence of restenosis. In 5 of 24 PTCA patients, MI or cardiac death occurred without any anginal warning. We were also impressed (during our chart reviews) with the difficulty experienced by the patients' primary physicians in identifying "anginal equivalents" post-PTCA for the reasons outlined in the Introduction section of this chapter. As argued earlier, this delay in the timely diagnosis of restenosis in dialysis patients may be poorly tolerated.

Marso *et al.* [54] retrospectively matched 23 hemodialysis patients with 44 control patients undergoing PTCA. Angina requiring hospitalization or AMI occurred in 63% of the dialysis patients and 20% of the controls within 6 months after PTCA. TVR occurred in 41% of dialysis patients and 11% of controls at 6 months. The AMI rate at 6 months post-PTCA was 23% for the dialysis patients and 0% for controls. At 6 months 13% of dialysis patients had died versus 2% of controls. At 3 years post-PTCA, 61% of dialysis patients and 11% of controls were dead. Seventy-five percent of the deaths in dialysis patients were attributable to cardiac causes.

Hang *et al.* [61] retrospectively studied 31 hemodialysis patients having PTCA in 1992–1996. There were 3 in-hospital deaths; clinical success was achieved in 28 patients (90%). Recurrent angina developed in 14 of 26 patients (54%) who were followed up. Ten of the 14 patients with angina were restudied, and all had restenosis at a prior PTCA vessel site. Of the 26 patients with postdischarge follow-up data, 11 (42%) died within 6 months and 17 (65%) died within 14 months. Ten of these 17 deaths (59%) were attributed to cardiovascular causes. No patients in this cohort underwent CAB after PTCA. This series is notable as it is one of the larger (in comparison to other papers) published single-center experiences of PTCA in dialysis patients, and for its abysmal outcome.

Sharma *et al.* [62] have reported preliminary data in 157 hemodialysis patients undergoing PCI in 1997–1999 (with stent use alone in 28% of patients and stents plus rotational atherectomy in 58% of patients). Glycoprotein IIb/IIIa inhibitors (i.e., abciximab) were used adjunctively in 76% of patients. An extraordinarily low post-PCI event rate was reported in this abstract: 24-month mortality of 14% (and 28% TVR). Confirmation of these preliminary findings would be extremely important, as this series from Mount Sinai Medical Center in New York presents a markedly more optimistic outcome for dialysis patients undergoing PCI in the modern interventional era. One intriguing aspect of this series is the large number of dialysis patients receiving glycoprotein IIb/IIIa inhibitors, as few data exist on the use of these agents in ESRD patients.

It should be apparent that the small sample size in most clinical studies hampers our understanding of PCI procedural outcomes in dialysis patients. Despite the inherent limitation of clinical registry data, there is much to be learned with large sample sizes. One interesting approach to data analysis is offered by Lacson and Ohno-Machado [63] in their use of "rough sets" and artificial neural nets to construct predictive models of major complications in patients with chronic renal failure undergoing

PTCA (using data from the New York State Angioplasty database). In their model, CHF and prior MI increased the risk of major periprocedural complications tenfold and 25-fold respectively.

PCI in nondialysis-dependent renal failure

Recent publications have highlighted the unfavorable outcome of patients with nondialysis-dependent CRF receiving PCI, and they suggest that the outcome of PCI in patients with nondialysis-dependent CRF may rival the poor results in dialysis patients.

Ting et al. [64] compared the outcome of 24 dialysis patients, 87 non-dialysis patients with serum Cr $\geq$ 3.0 mg/dL (CRF) and 2539 "control" patients with serum Cr < 3.0 mg/dL undergoing PCI in 1993–1996 at the Mayo Clinic. Unfortunately, patients who died in hospital were excluded from the survival analysis, as were those with procedural complications. Stents were used in 42% of the control group, 54% of the CRF group, and 54% of the dialysis patients. The estimated 2-year mortality was 5.6% for the control group, 30.4% for the CRF group, and 43.7% for the dialysis group in patients discharged alive without periprocedural complications. The contribution of radiocontrast-mediated acute renal failure to the mortality of patients with severe nondialysis-dependent CRF in this series is unknown.

The occurrence of elevated creatine kinase-MB (CK-MB) fraction elevation after successful PCI in patients with nondialysis-dependent renal failure is associated with adverse survival [65]. Gruberg et al. reported a 35.4% 1-year mortality in 70 patients with postprocedural CK-MB of >3X normal, 22.0% 1-year mortality in 72 patients with post-PCI CK-MB 1–3X normal, and 16.7% 1-year mortality in 184 patients without CK-MB rise. Increased serum levels of cardiac biomarkers (e.g., troponin I) after PCI in nonrenal patients may identify patients at higher risk for cardiac events [66], but there are few comparable data in patients with renal failure.

A notable clinical paper on PCI in renal failure is the work of Rubenstein et al. [49] at the Massachusetts General Hospital (Boston, MA) comparing the immediate and long-term outcomes of 362 renal failure patients (Cr > 1.5, median Cr = 1.9) and 2972 patients with normal renal function undergoing PCI in 1994–1997. Stents were used in 31.5% of the renal failure patients and 36.4% of nonrenal patients. The survival of an age- and gender-matched subset of the nonrenal patients was compared to the renal failure patients. Angiographically, the major difference in distribution of lesion types was the 17.3% type C lesions in the renal group versus 10.0% in the matched controls. The in-hospital mortality was 10.8% for the renal patients and 1.1% in the matched controls (p <0.0001). Blood transfusion

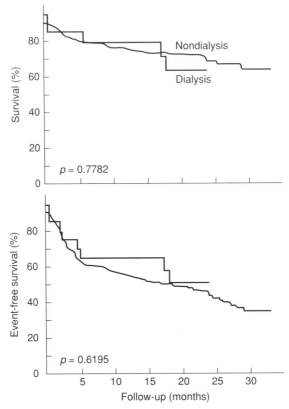

Figure 5 Kaplan–Meier survival curves (top) and Kaplan–Meier event-free survival (death, AMI, or repeat coronary revascularization curves) (bottom) of dialysis versus nondialysis patients within renal population. (From reference [49], with permission.)

occurred in 43.1% of the renal patients versus 13.8% of controls. The renal group included 27 dialysis patients, and their in-hospital mortality (11.1%) was identical to the nondialysis-dependent renal failure patients (10.8%). The 1-year actuarial survival was 75% for the renal failure group and 97% for the matched controls (p <0.00001). The event-free survival for death, AMI, or repeat coronary revascularization was 55% for the renal group and 78% for the matched controls (p <0.00001). As shown in Figure 5, the long-term survival of the dialysis subset, however, was not different than the other renal failure patients.

Gruberg *et al.* [56] have reported similar findings to Rubenstein *et al.* [49]. They retrospectively identified 9125 patients with normal renal function, 786 patients with chronic renal failure Cr $\geq$ 1.8 mg/dL and 95 patients with ESRD undergoing PCI in 1994–1997. About half of the patients in each group received stents. At 1-year follow-up the mortality was 48.8%

in the ESRD group, 25.7% in the CRF group, and 5.5% in the nonrenal cohort. Although diabetes was disproportionately represented in patients with renal failure (62.4% of ESRD, 47.9% of CRF, and 28.4% of the nonrenal group), in multivariate analysis dialysis (odds ratio 3.69; CI = 1.89–7.23) and CRF (odds ratio 1.74; CI = 1.20–2.51) were independently associated with increased death risk. One odd aspect of this report is the unusually high rate of periprocedural non-Q-wave MI (defined as a CK-MB elevation at least five times above the upper normal value without new Q-waves) in each subgroup: 17.6% of ESRD patients, 19.0% of CRF patients, and 13.8% of the nonrenal group. In the multivariate model, periprocedural non-Q-wave MI was strongly associated with late mortality (odds ratio 2.24; CI = 1.66–3.02). The cause of the high periprocedural non-Q-wave MI rate is not explored in this report, and the authors did not provide information on the absolute percentage of patients in each group receiving atheroablative procedures. One plausible explanation for the high periprocedure MI rates would be the utilization of atheroablative techniques. It is tempting to implicate the possible relation of a high periprocedural MI rate to the unexpectedly high mortality in the ESRD patients in this series, given the vulnerability of ESRD patients to sudden cardiac death.

Gruberg *et al.* [67], using the same database noted above, reported on 554 patients with nondialysis-dependent chronic renal failure (Cr = 1.4–3.0; mean Cr = 1.77 ± 0.35) receiving stents and retrospectively compared their outcome to 4530 stent patients with normal renal function. Despite similar angiographic lesion characteristics and high "procedural success" of 99% in both groups, the 1-year mortality was 17.4% in the renal failure group and 5.1% in the normal renal function group. Cardiac death accounted for 62% of all-cause death in both groups. In this series, 40.6% of the renal failure patients had diabetes, versus 23.7% in the normal renal function group. On multivariable analysis, diabetes and renal failure were both independently associated with a twofold increase in long-term death risk. Interestingly, the risk of TLR was *not* higher for patients with renal failure (again raising the issue of competing death risk).

A publication by Best *et al.* [57] demonstrates that there is a progressive gradient of risk associated with the severity of chronic renal failure in patients undergoing PCI. Using the Mayo Clinic interventional registry, they retrospectively analyzed the outcome of 5327 patients having PCI in 1994–1999. Patients were grouped by estimated creatinine clearance (>70, 50–69, 30–49, <30 mL/min and dialysis). Compared to a reference group of patients with estimated creatinine clearance of 90 mL/min, the risk ratio for long-term mortality after successful PCI for CrCl of 70 was 1.46 (95%CI 1.3–1.6), 2.25 (95%CI 1.8– 2.9) for CrCl of 50, 3.70 (95%CI 2.5–5.5) for CrCl

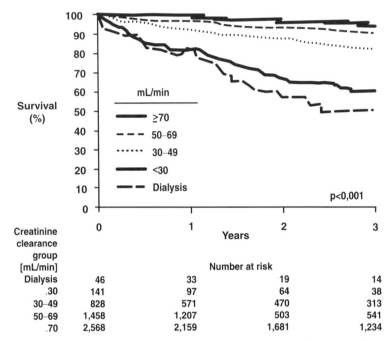

Figure 6 All-cause mortality after successful percutaneous coronary intervention in patients, based on their estimated creatinine clearance. (From reference [57], with permission.)

of 30, and 8.91 (95%CI 5.3–15.0) for dialysis patients. Figure 6 shows the estimated all-cause survival of the five patient groups and gradient of mortality risk associated with varying degrees of severity of chronic renal failure. Szczech *et al.* [68] have independently confirmed the additional mortality risk of chronic kidney disease in patients enrolled in the BARI study.

Acute renal failure complicating PCI in patients with preexistent chronic renal insufficiency is associated with very poor outcomes; particularly, if acute dialysis is required [69–72]. Gruberg *et al.* [69] studied 439 nondialysis-dependent patients with baseline $Cr \geq 1.8$ mg/dL undergoing PCI. In 161 patients with serum Cr rising $\geq 25\%$ within 48 hours after PCI or requiring dialysis, the 1-year mortality was 37.7% (vs 19.4% in patients without acute deterioration in renal function, $p = 0.001$). Of these 161 patients, 31 required acute dialysis, which was associated with a 22.6% in-hospital mortality and a 1-year 45.2% mortality. In a subsequent publication, Gruberg *et al.* [71] detailed the outcome of 51 patients (including 31 patients with baseline serum $Cr \geq 1.8$) requiring acute dialysis after PCI. The in-hospital mortality was 27.5% and 1-year mortality was 54.5%.

Gruberg *et al.* attributed contrast-induced nephrotoxicity as the etiology of acute renal failure in the majority of their patients, but the actual mechanism responsible for the increased mortality is speculative.

A panoply of therapies has been advanced for the prevention of contrast-induced nephropathy (a subject requiring its own entire book chapter). Some recent approaches include theophylline [73], forced diuresis [74], acetylcysteine [75], and fenoldopam [76,77] in combination with adequate preprocedure hydration and use of iso-osmolar contrast media. The use of combination therapy (fenoldopam and acetylcysteine) is intellectually appealing (due to potentially different protective effects), but is currently unproven. Clinical trial data have not supported the use of fenoldopam. Recent reviews by Pannu *et al.* and Barrett [77a, b] are recommended for a current perspective.

PCI vesus CAB

The interpretation of single-center studies is limited by the small sample sizes comprising the PTCA and CAB groups in their comparative analyses. All published data on PCI versus surgery in ESRD patients have been limited by retrospective study design, raising the possibility of selection bias confounding survival comparisons of different treatment groups. Three large cohort studies (of which two are currently published) have compared the outcome of dialysis patients undergoing PCI to CAB. Papers by Herzog *et al.* [52] and Szczech *et al.* [50] are published comparisons of the survival of dialysis patients following CAB or PTCA. The paper by Herzog *et al.* [53] is a preliminary analysis of comparative survival of dialysis patients after PTCA, coronary stents, and CAB (including the impact of internal mammary grafting).

Herzog *et al.* [52] published a retrospective survival analysis utilizing USRDS data of dialysis patients hospitalized for their first coronary revascularization procedure after ESRD initiation. There were 6887 patients receiving PTCA (1986–1995) and 7419 having CAB (1978–1995). The in-hospital mortality was 5.4% for the PTCA patients and 12.5% for CAB. The 2-year event-free survival (±SE) of PTCA patients was 52.9 ±0.7% for all-cause death, 72.5 ±0.7% for cardiac death, 81.2 ±0.6% for AMI, and 62.0% ±0.7% for the combined endpoint of cardiac death or AMI. In CAB patients, the comparable survivals were 56.9 ±0.6%, 75.8 ±0.6%, 91.9 ±0.4%, and 71.3 ±0.6%. In a comorbidity-adjusted Cox proportional hazards model, the relative risk of CAB surgery (vs PTCA) was 0.91 (95%CI 0.86–0.97), cardiac death 0.85(95%CI 0.78–0.92), AMI 0.37 (95%CI 0.32–0.45) and cardiac death or AMI 0.69 (95%CI 0.64–0.74). The risk of cardiac death was also analyzed by diabetic status. In diabetic patients, there was a 22% lower risk of cardiac death after CAB surgery (RR = 0.78; 95%CI 0.68–0.89) performed in 1990–1995 compared to PTCA performed in the same time period. In nondiabetic patients, there was a 10% lower risk of cardiac death after CAB surgery compared to PTCA in 1990–1995 (RR = 0.897; 95%CI 0.806–0.998). This finding of a larger relative survival improvement in a diabetic subgroup after CAB is consistent with other published data in nonrenal patients, notably the BARI study.

The survival advantage associated with CAB (versus PTCA) in dialysis patients is statistically evident at 6 months after revascularization in the data of Herzog *et al.* This point is noteworthy, as the short-term survival (e.g., ≤90 days) of dialysis patients undergoing PCI is actually more favorable than surgery. Thus, PCI (including PTCA) may be appropriate for selected short-term palliative indications. As alluded to in the Introduction of this chapter, it is plausible that clinically inapparent restenosis may be contributing to the excess deaths after PCI, and surveillance stress imaging (or angiography) could improve the outcome after PCI.

There are obvious limitations to the data of Herzog *et al.*; the most important ones are the retrospective study design and biased selection for a particular revascularization procedure. It could be argued that there are inherent clinical differences in the PTCA and CAB groups making survival comparisons after revascularization difficult; particularly, if intrinsically "healthier" patients received surgery (i.e., selection bias). The paper by Szczech *et al.* [50] presents an opposite conclusion that Herzog *et al.* underestimated the survival advantage of CAB, because the USRDS database does not include clinical data such as ejection fraction or presence of left main coronary disease. Using New York State clinical databases, Szczech *et al.* compared the outcome of 244 ESRD patients undergoing CAB and 163 ESRD patients with PCI (essentially PTCA). Their analysis was strengthened by comparing subgroups of patients with varying degrees of CAD severity that were not characterized by "unbalanced" procedure utilization (i.e., if one treatment strategy was utilized <10% of the time, the patients in the subgroup were excluded from analysis). The adjusted estimated 2-year survival was 51.9% after PCI and 77.4% after CAB. In a Cox model, the risk of death was 61% lower after CAB versus PCI ($p = 0.0006$). It is possible, however, that Szczech *et al.* have overestimated the survival advantage of CAB in dialysis patients due to the relatively small sample size of ESRD patients in the New York state cardiac surgery and angioplasty registries (<3% of the sample size reported by Herzog *et al.* in their USRDS studies).

The survival of dialysis patients after PTCA, coronary stents, and CAB has been one major area of interest of the Cardiovascular Special Studies

Center of USRDS. Herzog *et al.* [53a] reported on the survival of 8724 dialysis patients hospitalized for CAB, 5470 patients received PTCA alone, and 7118 patients received coronary stents in 1995–1999. The impact of internal mammary grafts in the surgery group was also evaluated. The 2-year survival of PTCA patients was 49.1%, 51.1% for patients receiving stents, 50.3% for CAB without internal mammary grafts, and 60.6% in the 5497 patients receiving internal mammary grafts. In a comorbidity-adjusted Cox model the risk of all-cause death was 9% lower for stent (p <0.0001), 10% lower for CAB ($p = 0.0003$) without internal mammary grafting, and 25% lower for CAB ($p < 0.0001$) with internal mammary grafting, compared to PTCA. The survival advantage of CAB in dialysis patients compared to PCI is predominantly associated with the use of internal mammary grafts, and appears to be present in both diabetic and nondiabetic ESRD.

There are a paucity of published data on the comparative survival of renal transplant recipients after coronary intervention, but we have presented preliminary data and published a paper on the survival of renal transplant recipients after PTCA, coronary artery stents, and CAB [78a]. We identified 1100 patients hospitalized for CAB (of whom 812 received internal mammary grafts), 652 for PTCA alone, and 909 received coronary stents in 1995–1999 using the USRDS database. The in-hospital death was 6.2% for CAB, 4.2% for PTCA, and 2.3% for the stent group. The estimated 2-year survival of the PTCA group was 81.6%, 82.5% for stent, and 80.6% for CAB. After adjustment for comorbidity, there was no difference in all-cause or cardiac survival in a Cox model for PTCA, stent, or CAB. There was, however, a 36% reduction in the risk of cardiac death or AMI for CAB and a 12% reduction in risk for the stent group compared to PTCA. It is apparent that the survival of renal transplant recipients is considerably better after coronary intervention than dialysis patients.

Adjunctive therapy with PCI in patients with ESRD

Role of heparin

Unfractionated heparin has been used almost uniformly in PCI studies. Physicians seem to be comfortable with the use of heparin partly because of its ease of delivery, shorter half-life and the ability to monitor activated clotting time (ACT) and activated PTT. Few data are available on the safety and efficacy of low molecular weight heparin in ESRD patients.

Role of direct thrombin inhibitors
Bivalirudin (angiomax)
Bivalirudin, a direct thrombin inhibitor, is predominantly renally excreted, and appropriate dose adjustments for all degrees of renal impairment,

including dialysis dependence, are provided by the manufacturer [79]. In the nonuremic population bivalirudin has been shown to improve the procedural success rate and reduce bleeding complications when compared to weight-adjusted heparin during PTCA [80].

Role of GP2b3a inhibitors

In the nonuremic patients, adjunctive therapy with glycoprotein IIb/IIIa inhibitors has reduced the incidence of stent thrombosis and improved outcomes [81,82]. In a Mayo clinic retrospective analysis of 230 patients receiving abciximab with creatinine clearance (CC) <50 mL/min and 367 patients with CC = 50–70 mL/min found no interaction between CC and death, MI or major bleeding, suggesting abciximab is safe and as efficacious in CRF patients as in nonuremic patients [83].

In contrast, Frilling *et al.* [84], using the Ludwigshafen IIb/IIIa-Antagonist Registry, reported on 44 patients with impaired renal function (Cr $\geq$ 1.3 mg/dL) and found a higher rate of major bleeding (4.5%) versus 0.6% in 996 nonrenal control patients ($p = 0.003$). In a multivariate analysis, there was a fivefold risk of any bleeding episode associated with abciximab (odds ratio 5.1; 95%CI 1.9–13.8).

Current U.S. product labeling of available glycoprotein IIb/IIIa inhibitors includes a reduced dose of eptifibatide in chronic renal failure patients (with no additional recommendation for Cr $\geq$ 4.0), reduction of tirofiban dose by 50% in dialysis patients, and no dose adjustment for abciximab. It must be stressed that there are currently few published data on safety or efficacy of these agents in dialysis patients. Prudence dictates careful clinical observation of dialysis patients following PCI, regardless of the particular therapeutic strategy employed.

Right heart monitoring

In our own institution, we have found that the use of periprocedure right heart monitoring is helpful for guiding post-PCI management. Although the universal use of very low osmolality agents in our lab (i.e., iodixanol) reduces the degree of postprocedure volume stress, the necessity for urgent dialysis/ultrafiltration (or alternatively, volume resuscitation/transfusion in the setting of occult massive retroperitoneal bleed) can be anticipated post-PCI with right heart monitoring.

Trends in newer therapy: brachytherapy and drug-eluting stents

The role of radiation as an adjunct to PCI is now established in the setting of in-stent restenosis in nonuremic patients [85–89]. The only published data in patients with CRF are from the Washington Hospital Center and no data are available in ESRD patients. Gruberg *et al.* [90] analyzed the data for in-stent restenosis treated with a mix of intracoronary gamma (192-iridium train source) radiation and beta (yttrium) radiation. They compared 118 CRF patients (mean serum creatinine of 2.0) with 481 nonrenal patients receiving intracoronary radiation and 14 CRF patients receiving placebo for treatment of in-stent restenosis in a retrospective analysis. A majority, but not all, had angiographic evaluation at 6 months for restenosis. Their results indicate that the re-restenosis rate in CRF patients treated with radiation was significantly lower at 6 months (22.6% vs 53.8%) than CRF patients treated with placebo. TVR was lower (23.7% vs 78.6%) as was TLR (15.3% vs 71.4%). Event-free survival was significantly better in the brachytherapy group (72.9% vs 21.4%) at 6 months. When compared to patients with normal renal function, brachytherapy seemed to be effective locally with comparable re-restenosis rates, TVR, TLR, and late total occlusion rates in the CRF population, but the overall mortality (7.6% vs 1.9%) and cardiac mortality (6.8% vs 1.5%) was significantly higher at 6 months in the CRF group. This study confirms the safety of intracoronary radiation therapy in CRF population and suggests that in-stent restenosis can be treated effectively in CRF patients.

The most currently promising advancement in PCI is the development of the drug-eluting stent. Preliminary data have suggested markedly reduced rates of in-stent restenosis [91–98]. Surprising results of the RAVEL trial, a randomized, double-blind comparison of 120 patients receiving sirolimus-coated Bx Velocity stents versus 118 patients with uncoated Bx Velocity stents for native coronary lesions, included a restenosis rate of 26.6% in the control group and 0% restenosis in the coated stent group at 6 months [98]. There are no data on drug-eluting stents in patients with renal failure (and RAVEL excluded some patients at high risk for restenosis). It is still speculative whether drug-eluting stents prevent or merely delay the onset of restenosis, but this new approach to PCI is an exciting prospect for the treatment of coronary artery disease in patients with renal failure.

Conclusion

It should be apparent that patients with renal failure are at high risk for cardiovascular morbidity and mortality after percutaneous coronary intervention (PCI). We have provided an overview of the relatively limited body of knowledge on PCI in renal failure, and clearly there are many potentially fruitful areas for future clinical investigation.

An interventional registry for PCI in renal failure (with special attention to ESRD) would provide therapy (e.g., device)-specific outcome data at relatively modest cost, and it would facilitate the design of large-scale clinical trials targeting patients with renal failure. A prospective study of PCI outcome in ESRD patients is sorely needed, as we still do not have an accurate estimation of restenosis rates after PCI in dialysis patients (and the accuracy of noninvasive detection of restenosis). Such a study would ideally include a prospective cohort of at least several hundred patients undergoing noninvasive stress imaging before angiography, quantitative coronary angiography, measurement of fractional flow reserve (and perhaps IVUS [intravascular ultrasound]) at the time of PCI, and importantly, repeat noninvasive stress imaging and quantitative coronary angiography (and IVUS) in *all* patients at restenosis-appropriate time intervals (e.g., 3–6 months) and at 1 year. In a more ambitious trial, promising therapies (such as drug-eluting stents) could be compared to "conventional" treatments.

Data pertaining to the safety and efficacy of standard adjunctive pharmacologic therapy are virtually nonexistent in ESRD patients. Outcome data on glycoprotein IIb/IIIa inhibitors would be an important part of the proposed interventional registry for PCI in renal failure, but clinical trials of these agents targeting patients with renal failure would be particularly desirable. The role of contrast-mediated nephropathy for adverse outcome and its prevention (perhaps with combination therapy including acetylcysteine and fenoldopam) is another potential area for clinical trials in patients with chronic renal failure.

Finally, there may be better alternatives to PCI for coronary revascularization in dialysis patients. The "ultimate" clinical trial may be a prospective comparison of PCI (perhaps drug-eluting stents and other effective adjunctive pharmacologic agents) and surgical coronary revascularization employing arterial conduits (and recent advances in surgical techniques, including "off-pump" CAB surgery). There may be other more "radical" approaches to dealing with the staggering cardiovascular mortality of ESRD patients. The majority of cardiac deaths in dialysis patients are attributed to a combination of unexpected sudden death and arrhythmias; devices targeting the prevention of arrhythmic death might have even a greater potential impact on survival. ESRD patients are a group at particularly high risk for suffering adverse cardiac outcomes, and they potentially will reap the largest benefit from effective strategies for the prevention, diagnosis, and treatment of cardiovascular disease.

References

1 *USRDS 2000 Annual Data Report*. NIH Publication No. 00-3176. National Institutes of Health, Bethesda, MD; 2000:589–684.
2 *USRDS 2000 Annual Data Report*. NIH Publication No. 00-3176. National Institute of Diabetes and Digestive and Kidney Diseases, Bethesda, MD; 2000:583–689.

3 *USRDS 2000 Annual Data Report*. NIH Publication No. 00-3176. National Institutes of Health, Bethesda, MD; 2000:69–75.

4 Jones CA, McQuillan GM, Kusek JW, *et al.* Serum creatinine levels in the US population: 3rd National Health and Nutrition Examination Survey. *Am J Kidney Dis* 1998;**32**(6):992–999.

5 Luke RG. Chronic renal failure—a vasculopathic state. *N Engl J Med* 1998;**339**(12):841–843.

6 Blacher J, Guerin AP, Pannier B, Marchais SJ, Safar ME, London GM. Impact of aortic stiffness on survival in end-stage renal disease. *Circulation* 1999;**99**:2434–2439.

7 Goodman WG, Goldin J, Kuizon BD, *et al.* Coronary-artery calcification in young adults with end-stage renal disease who are undergoing dialysis. *N Engl J Med* 2000;**342**(20):1478–1483.

8 Miyazaki H, Matsuoka H, Itabe H, *et al.* Hemodialysis impairs endothelial function via oxidative stress: effects of vitamin E-coated dialyzer. *Circulation* 2000;**101**(9):1002–1006.

9 Manske CL. Hyperglycemia and intensive glycemic control in diabetic patients with chronic renal disease. *Am J Kidney Dis* 1998;**32**(5, suppl. 3):S157–S171.

10 Schwarz U, Amann K, Ritz E. Why are coronary plaques more malignant in the uratemic patient? *Nephrol Dial Transplant* 1999;**14**(1):224–225.

11 Schwarz U, Buzello M, Ritz E, *et al.* Morphology of coronary atherosclerotic lesions in patients with end-stage renal failure. *Nephrol Dial Transplant* 2000;**15**(2):218–223.

12 Tamashiro M, Iseki K, Sunagawa O, *et al.* Significant association between the progression of coronary artery calcification and dyslipidemia in patients on chronic hemodialysis. *Am J Kidney Dis* 2001;**38**(1):64–69.

13 Amann K, Rychlik I, Miltenberger-Milteny G, Ritz E. Left ventricular hypertrophy in renal failure. *Kidney Int Suppl* 1998;**68**:S78–S85.

14 Amann K, Ritz E. Cardiac disease in chronic uremia: pathophysiology. *Adv Ren Replace Ther* 1997;**4**(3):212–224.

15 Ritz E, Amann K, Tornig J, Schwarz U, Stein G. Some cardiac abnormalities in renal failure. In: *Advances in Nephrology*. Mosby-Year Book, Philadelphia; 1998:85–103.

16 Amann K, Buzello M, Simonaviciene A, *et al.* Capillary/myocyte mismatch in the heart in renal failure—a role for erythropoietin? *Nephrol Dial Transplant* 2000;**15**(7):964–969.

17 Bleyer AJ, Russell GB, Satko SG. Sudden and cardiac death rates in hemodialysis patients. *Kidney Int* 1999;**55**:1553–1559.

18 Ma JZ, Collins AJ, Herzog CA. Survival of dialysis patients sustaining acute myocardial infarction (AMI): hemodialysis (HD) vs. peritoneal dialysis (PD). *J Am Soc Nephrol* 1999;**10**:248A.

19 Herzog CA, Ma JZ, Collins AJ. Poor long-term survival after acute myocardial infarction among patient on long-term dialysis. *N Engl J Med* 1998;**339**:799–805.

20 Chertow GM, Normand ST, Silva LR, McNeil BJ. Survival after acute myocardial infarction in patients with end-stage renal disease: results from the cooperative cardiovascular project. *Am J Kidney Dis* 2000;**35**:1044–1051.

21 Iseki K, Fukiyama K. Long-term prognosis and incidence of acute myocardial infarction in patients on chronic hemodialysis. The Okinawa Dialysis Study Group. *Am J Kidney Dis* 2000;**36**(4):820–825.

22 Beattie JN, Soman SS, Sandberg KR, *et al.* Determinants of mortality after

myocardial infarction in patients with advanced renal dysfunction. *Am J Kidney Dis* 2001;**37**(6):1191–1200.

23 Herzog CA. Acute myocardial infarction in patients with end-stage renal disease. *Kidney Int* 1999;**56**(suppl. 71):S130–S133.

24 Herzog CA, Ma JZ, Collins AJ. Long-term survival of dialysis patients receiving thrombolytic therapy for acute myocardial infarction in the United States. *Circulation* 1999;**100**(suppl. I):I-304.

25 Wright RS, Albright R, Dvorak D, *et al.* Renal dysfunction and acute myocardial infarction: increasing risk of mortality parallels degree of renal dysfunction. *J Am Soc Nephrol* 2001;**12**:89A.

26 Dierkes J, Domrose U, Westphal S, *et al.* Cardiac troponin T predicts mortality in patients with end-stage renal disease. *Circulation* 2000;**102**(16):1964–1969.

27 Herzog CA, Murakami MM, Davis GK, *et al.* Prognostic value of cardiac troponin testing in end stage renal disease. *J Am Soc Nephrol* 2000;**11**:272A.

28 Kasiske BL. Epidemiology of cardiovascular disease after renal transplantation. *Transplantation* 2001;**72**(suppl. 6):S5–S8.

29 Kasiske BL, Ramos EL, Gaston RS, *et al.* The evaluation of renal transplant candidates: clinical practice guidelines. *J Am Soc Nephrol* 1995;**6**:1–34.

30 Herzog CA. Acute MI in dialysis patients: how can we improve the outlook. *J Crit Illness* 1999;**14**:613–621.

31 Herzog CA, Marwick TH, Pheley AM, White CW, Rao VK, Dick CD. Dobutamine stress echocardiography for the detection of significant coronary artery disease in renal transplant candidates. *Am J Kidney Dis* 1999;**33**(6):1080–1090.

32 Herzog CA. Diagnosis and treatment of ischemic heart disease in dialysis patients. *Curr Opin Nephrol Hypertens* 1997;**6**(6):558–565.

33 Herzog CA. Noninvasive diagnosis of CAD in patients with end-stage renal disease. In: Marwick TH, ed. *Cardiac Stress Testing and Imaging: A Clinician's Guide*.: Churchill Livingstone, New York; 1996:203–222.

34 Herzog C, Huiras BE, Bart BA. Are nuclear myocardial perfusion and echocardiography (ECHO) stress imaging studies equivalent in the assessment of coronary artery disease in patients with end stage renal disease? *J Am Soc Nephrol* 2001;**12**:383A.

35 Manske CL, Wang Y, Rector TS, Wilson RF, White CW. Coronary revascularization in insulin-dependent diabetic patients with chronic renal failure. *Lancet* 1992;**340**:998–1002.

36 Herzog C, Ma J, Collins A. Repeat coronary revascularization rates after angioplasty, stenting, bypass surgery and competing death risk in dialysis patients. *Circulation* 2001;**104**(17):II-424.

37 Ma JZ, *et al.* The likelihood of repeated coronary revascularization procedures (CRP) after first CRP in dialysis patients. *J Am Soc Nephrol* 1999;**10**:249A.

38 National Kidney Foundation Task Force on Cardiovascular Disease. Controlling the epidemic of cardiovascular disease in chronic renal disease: What do we know? What do we need to know? Where do we go from here? Special report from the National Kidney Foundation Task Force on Cardiovascular Disease. *Am J Kidney Dis* 1998;**32**:S1–S199.

39 Asinger RW, Henry TD, Herzog CA, Paulsen PR, Kane RL. Clinical outcomes of

PTCA in chronic renal failure: a case-control study for comorbid features and evaluation of dialysis dependence. *J Invasive Cardiol* 2001;**13**(1):21–28.

40 Agirbasli M, Weintraub WS, Chang GL, *et al.* Outcome of coronary revascularization in patients on renal dialysis. *Am J Cardiol* 2000;**86**(4):395–399.

41 Le Feuvre C, Dambrin G, Helft G, *et al.* Clinical outcome following coronary angioplasty in dialysis patients: a case-control study in the era of coronary stenting. *Heart* 2001;**85**:556–560.

42 Azar RR, Prpic R, Ho KK, *et al.* Impact of end-stage renal disease on clinical and angiographic outcomes after coronary stenting. *Am J Cardiol* 2000;**86**(5):485–489.

43 Ohmoto Y, Ayabe M, Hara K, *et al.* Long-term outcome of percutaneous transluminal coronary angioplasty and coronary artery bypass grafting in patients with end-stage renal disease. *Jpn Circ J* 1999;**63**(12):981–987.

44 Simsir SA, Kohlman-Trigoboff D, Flood R, Lindsay J, Smith BM. A comparison of coronary artery bypass grafting and percutaneous transluminal coronary angioplasty in patients on hemodialysis. *Cardiovasc Surg* 1998;**6**(5):500–505.

45 Koyanagi T, Nishida H, Kitamura M, *et al.* Comparison of clinical outcomes of coronary artery bypass grafting and percutaneous transluminal coronary angioplasty in renal dialysis patients. *Ann Thorac Surg* 1996;**61**:1793–1796.

46 Rinehart A, Herzog C, Collins A, Flack J, Ma J, Opsahl J. A comparison of coronary angioplasty and coronary artery bypass grafting outcomes in chronic dialysis patients. *Am J Kidney Dis* 1995;**25**(2):281–290.

47 Takeshita S, Isshiki T, Tagawa H, Yamaguchi T. Percutaneous transluminal coronary angioplasty for chronic dialysis patients. *J Invasive Cardiol* 1993;**5**:345–350.

48 Kahn JK, Rutherford BD, McConahay DR, Johnson WL, Giorgi LV, Hartzler GO. Short- and long-term outcome of percutaneous transluminal coronary angioplasty in chronic dialysis patients. *Am Heart J* 1990;**119**:484–489.

49 Rubenstein MH, Harrell LC, Sheynberg BV, Schunkert H, Bazari H, Palacios IF. Are patients with renal failure good candidates for percutaneous coronary revascularization in the new device era? *Circulation* 2000;**102**(24):2966–2972.

50 Szczech L, Reddan D, Owen W, Jr, *et al.* Differential survival after coronary revascularization procedures among patients with renal insufficiency. *Kidney Int* 2001;**60**:292–299.

51 Ahmed WH, Shubrooks SJ, Gibson M, Baim DS , Bittl JA. Complications and long-term outcome after percutaneous coronary angioplasty in chronic hemodialysis patients. *Am Heart J* 1994;**128**:252–255.

52 Herzog C, Ma J, Collins A. Long-term outcome of dialysis patients in the United States with coronary revascularization procedures. *Kidney Int* 1999;**56**:324–332.

53 Herzog C, Ma J, Collins A. Long term survival of dialysis patients in the US after coronary angioplasty, coronary artery stenting, and coronary artery bypass surgery. *Circulation* 2001;**104**(17): II-704.

53a Herzog CA, Ma JZ, Collins AJ: Comparative survival of dialysis patients in the United States after coronary angioplasty, coronary artery stenting, and coronary artery bypass graft surgery and impact of diabetes. *Circulation* 2002;**106**:2207–2211.

54 Marso SP, Gimple LW, Philbrick JT, DiMarco JP. Effectiveness of percutaneous coronary interventions to prevent recurrent coronary events in patients on chronic hemodialysis. *Am J Cardiol* 1998;**82**:378–380.

55 Schoebel FC, Gradaus F, Ivens K, *et al.* Restenosis after elective coronary balloon angioplasty in patients with end stage renal disease: a case-control study using quantitative coronary angiography. *Heart* 1997;**78**:337–342.

56 Gruberg L, Dangas G, Mehran R, *et al.* Clinical outcome following percutaneous coronary interventions in patients with chronic renal failure. *Catheter Cardiovasc Interv* 2002;**55**(1):66–72.

57 Best PJ, Lennon R, Ting HH, *et al.* The impact of renal insufficiency on clinical outcomes in patients undergoing percutaneous coronary interventions. *J Am Coll Cardiol* 2002;**39**(7):1113–1119.

58 Le Feuvre C, Dambrin G, Helft G, *et al.* Comparison of clinical outcome following coronary stenting or balloon angioplasty in dialysis versus non-dialysis patients. *Am J Cardiol* 2000;**85**(11):1365–1368.

59 Reusser LM, Osborn LA, White HJ, Sexson R, Crawford MH. Increased morbidity after coronary angioplasty in patients on chronic hemodialysis. *Am J Cardiol* 1994;**73**:965–967.

60 Kober G, Vallbracht C, Giesecke R, Grutzmacher P, Fassbinder W, Kaltenbach M. Transluminal coronary angioplasty in patients with chronic kidney failure. *Dtsch Med Wochenschr* 1985;**110**(4):129–134.

61 Hang CL, Chen MC, Wu BJ, Wu CJ, Chua S, Fu M. Short- and long-term outcomes after percutaneous transluminal coronary angioplasty in chronic hemodialysis patients. *Catheter Cardiovasc Interv* 1999;**47**(4):430–433.

62 Sharma SK, Cheema AM, Andrews P, *et al.* Current status of percutaneous coronary intervention (PCI) in patients with chronic renal failure on hemodialysis. *Circulation* 2000;**102**(18):II-480.

63 Lacson RC, Ohno-Machado L. Major complications after angioplasty in patients with chronic renal failure: a comparison of predictive models. *Proc AMIA Symp* 2000;457–461.

64 Ting H, Takirkheli N, Berger P, *et al.* Evaluation of long-term survival after successful percutaneous coronary intervention among patients with chronic renal failure. *Am J Cardiol* 2001;**87**(5):630–633.

65 Gruberg L, Mehran R, Waksman R, *et al.* Creatine kinase-MB fraction elevation after percutaneous coronary intervention in patients with chronic renal failure. *Am J Cardiol* 2001;**87**(12):1356–1360.

66 Cantor WJ, Newby LK, Christenson RH, *et al.* Elevated troponin-I after percutaneous coronary intervention is a powerful prognostic indicator. *Circulation* 2000;**102**(18):II-753.

67 Gruberg L, Weissman NJ, Waksman R, *et al.* Comparison of outcomes after percutaneous coronary revascularization with stents in patients with and without mild chronic renal insufficiency. *Am J Cardiol* 2002;**89**(1):54–57.

68 Szczech LA, Best PJ, Crowley E, *et al.* Outcomes of patients with chronic renal insufficiency in the bypass angioplasty revascularization investigation. *Circulation* 2002;**105**(19):2253–2258.

69 Gruberg L, Mintz GS, Mehran R, *et al.* The prognostic implications of further renal function deterioration within 48 h of interventional coronary procedures in patients with pre-existent chronic renal insufficiency. *J Am Coll Cardiol* 2000;**36**(5):1542–1548.

70 McCullough PA, Wolyn R, Rocher LL, Levin RN, O'Neill WW. Acute renal failure after coronary intervention: incidence, risk factors, and relationship to mortality. *Am J Med* 1997;**103**(5):368–375.

71 Gruberg L, Mehran R, Dangas G, *et al.* Acute renal failure requiring dialysis after percutaneous coronary interventions. *Catheter Cardiovasc Interv* 2001;**52**(4):409–416.

72 Rihal CS, Textor SC, Grill DE, *et al.* Incidence and prognostic importance of acute renal failure after percutaneous coronary intervention. *Circulation* 2002;**105**(19):2259–2264.

73 Erley CM, Duda SH, Rehfuss D, *et al.* Prevention of radiocontrast-media-induced nephropathy in patients with pre-existing renal insufficiency by hydration in combination with the adenosine antagonist theophylline. *Nephrol Dial Transplant* 1999;**14**(5):1146–1149.

74 Stevens MA, McCullough PA, Tobin KJ, *et al.* A prospective randomized trial of prevention measures in patients at high risk for contrast nephropathy: results of the PRINCE Study. Prevention of radiocontrast induced nephropathy clinical evaluation. *J Am Coll Cardiol* 1999;**33**(2):403–411.

75 Tepel M, van der GM, Schwarzfeld C, Laufer U, Liermann D, Zidek W. Prevention of radiographic-contrast-agent-induced reductions in renal function by acetylcysteine. *N Engl J Med* 2000;**343**(3):180–184.

76 Tumlin JA, Murray PT, Mathur VS, Wang A. A multicenter, double-blind, placebo-controlled trial of fenoldopam mesylate in the prevention of radiocontrast nephropathy in patients with moderate to severe renal insufficiency. *J Am Soc Nephrol* 2000;**11**:135A.

77 Kini AS, Mitre CA, Kamran M, *et al.* Changing trends in incidence and predictors of radiographic contrast nephropathy after percutaneous coronary intervention with use of fenoldopam. *Am J Cardiol* 2002;**89**(8):999–1002.

77a Pannu N, Wiebe N, Tonelli M, Prophylaxis strategies for contrast-induced nephropathy. *JAMA* 2006;**295**:2765–2779.

77b Barrett BJ, Parfrey PS, Preventing nephropathy induced by contrast medium. *N Engl J Med* 2006;**354**:379–86.

78 Herzog CA, Ma JZ, Collins AJ. Long-term outcome of renal transplant recipients in the US after coronary artery bypass surgery, coronary angioplasty, and coronary stenting. *Circulation* 2001;**104**(17):II-704.

78a Herzog CA, Ma JZ, Collins AJ. Long-term outcome of renal transplant recipients in the United States after coronary revascularization procedure. *Circulation.* 2004;**109**(23):2866–2871.

79 Robson R. The use of bivalirudin in patients with renal impairment. *J Invasive Cardiol* 2000;**12**(suppl. F):33F.

80 Bittl JA, Feit F. A randomized comparison of bivalirudin and heparin in patients undergoing coronary angioplasty for postinfarction angina. Hirulog Angioplasty Study Investigators. *Am J Cardiol* 1998;**82**(8B):49P.

81 Kereiakes DJ, Lincoff AM, Miller DP, *et al.* Abciximab therapy and unplanned coronary stent deployment: favorable effects on stent use, clinical outcomes, and bleeding complications. EPILOG Trial Investigators. *Circulation* 1998;**97**(9):857–864.

82 The RESTORE Investigators. Effects of platelet glycoprotein IIb/IIIa blockade with tirofiban on adverse cardiac events in patients with unstable angina or acute myocardial infarction undergoing coronary angioplasty. Randomized efficacy study of tirofiban for outcomes and restenosis. *Circulation* 1997;**96**(5):1445–1453.

83 Best PJM, Lennon R, Ting HH, *et al.* The safety of abciximab before percutaneous coronary revascularization in patients with chronic renal insufficiency. *J Am Coll Cardiol* 2001;**37**(2):4A.

84 Frilling B, Zahn R, Fraiture B, *et al.* Comparison of efficacy and complication rates after percutaneous coronary interventions in patients with and without renal insufficiency treated with abciximab. *Am J Cardiol* 2002;**89**(4):450–452.

85 Leon MB, Teirstein PS, Moses JW, *et al.* Localized intracoronary gamma-radiation therapy to inhibit the recurrence of restenosis after stenting. *N Engl J Med* 2001;**344**(4):250–256.

86 Teirstein PS, Massullo V, Jani S, *et al.* Two-year follow-up after catheter-based radiotherapy to inhibit coronary restenosis. *Circulation* 1999;**99**:243–247.

87 Teirstein PS, Massullo V, Jani S, *et al.* Catheter-based radiotherapy to inhibit restenosis after coronary stenting. *N Engl J Med* 1997;**336**:1697–703.

88 Teirstein PS, Massullo V, Jani S, *et al.* Three-year clinical and angiographic follow-up after intracoronary radiation: results of a randomized clinical trial. *Circulation* 2000;**101**(4):360–365.

89 Verin V, Popowski Y, De Bruyne B, *et al.* Endoluminal beta-radiation therapy for the prevention of coronary restenosis after balloon angioplasty. *N Engl J Med* 2001;**344**(4):243–249.

90 Gruberg L, Waksman R, Ajani AE, *et al.* The effect of intracoronary radiation for the treatment of recurrent in-stent restenosis in patients with chronic renal failure. *J Am Coll Cardiol* 2001;**38**(4):1049–1053.

91 Sousa JE, Costa MA, Abizaid AC, *et al.* Sustained suppression of neointimal proliferation by sirolimus-eluting stents: one-year angiographic and intravascular ultrasound follow-up. *Circulation* 2001;**104**(17):2007–2011.

92 Sousa JE, Costa MA, Abizaid A, *et al.* Lack of neointimal proliferation after implantation of sirolimus-coated stents in human coronary arteries: a quantitative coronary angiography and three-dimensional intravascular ultrasound study. *Circulation* 2001;**103**(2):192–195.

93 Sousa JE, Morice MC, Serruys PW, *et al.* The RAVEL Study: a randomized study with the sirolimus coated BX velocity balloon-expandable stent in the treatment of patients with de novo native coronary artery lesions. *Circulation* 2001;**104**(17):II-463.

94 Sousa JE, Abizaid A, Abizaid A, *et al.* First human experience with sirolimus coated Bx VELOCITY stent: clinical, angiographic and ultrasound late results. *Circulation* 2000;**102**(18, suppl. II):815.

95 Grube E, Silber SM, Hauptman KE. Taxus I: prospective, randomized, double-blind comparison of NIRx stents coated with paclitaxel in a polymer carrier in de-novo coronary lesions compared with uncoated controls. *Circulation* 2001;**104**(17):II-463.

96 Rensing B, Vos J, Smiths P, *et al.* Coronary restenosis prevention with a rapamycin coated stent. *J Am Coll Cardiol* 2001;**37**(2, suppl. A):47A.

97 Feres F, Costa MA, Abizaid A, *et al.* Comparison between sirolimus-coated and non-coated stent implantation in human coronary arteries. *J Am Coll Cardiol* 2001;**37**(2, suppl. A):47A.

98 Morice MC, Serruys PW, Sousa JE, *et. al.* A randomized comparison of a sirolimus-eluting stent with a standard stent for coronary revascularization. *N Engl J Med* 2002;**346**(23):1773–1780.

Cardiopulmonary bypass in patients with chronic renal failure: techniques and management

Michael A. Sobieski II, Mark S. Slaughter

Introduction

The complex hemodynamic and physiologic changes which occur while the patient is supported by cardiopulmonary bypass (CPB) is further complicated by the presence of chronic renal failure (CRF). "These patients present extraordinary problems not only medically and surgically, but philosophically" [1] as noted by Dr Allan Lansing in 1968. The CRF patient can present with a multitude of medical problems such as chronic anemia, pulmonary edema, electrolyte and acid/base imbalance, and decreased protein levels. These associated medical issues are all due to the disease process itself or the treatment of CRF. It has been documented that careful perioperative management of this select subgroup of cardiovascular patients has a direct impact on a successful operative outcome [2,3].

There have been a modest number of reports in the literature addressing the issues related to CPB in the CRF patient. The majority have focused on the CPB phase of the operation [1–25]. It is during this period of cardiac surgery when pump flow and perfusion pressure are under complete control by the operative team. The perioperative period during cardiopulmonary support provides an excellent opportunity to implement a comprehensive management plan. Careful cooperation and communication between the surgeon, anesthesiologist, and perfusionist are essential to achieve the best possible outcome.

Preoperative evaluation

A good preoperative plan begins with a careful assessment of the patient presenting for surgery. In addition to CRF, studies have demonstrated other risk factors such as age, smoking, diabetes, and left ventricular ejection fraction, which are independent predictors of late mortality in this group of patients [4]. All factors normally evaluated for patients undergoing cardiovascular surgery are assessed at this time with special attention to those components that can be altered to improve outcomes.

Fluid status

CRF patients undergoing elective cardiac surgery usually arrive at the operating room in a normovolemic state due to their routine hemodialysis within 24 hours prior to surgery. Sometimes, adequate preoperative hemodialysis is not possible due to angina from critical coronary artery disease or hypotension from rapid fluid shifts in patients with valvular heart disease. In urgent or emergent cases or those patients unable to undergo their routine dialysis preoperatively, attempts should be made to determine their current fluid status. Information such as intake and output over the previous 24-hour period and baseline filling pressures (right atrium and pulmonary artery) obtained upon insertion of the Swan–Ganz catheter are critical for intraoperative management. Additionally, assessment of the skin for normal turgor and the extremities for peripheral edema will aid in determining the patient's fluid status. It is also common for the CRF patient to have an associated anemic condition. While not all CRF patients are symptomatic due to the compensatory mechanisms associated with chronic anemia [2,5], it is necessary to maintain a hemoglobin level of 7–8 g per 100 mL of blood volume. This is important to insure sufficient oxygen carrying capacity and perfusion at the cellular level.

Electrolyte status

Abnormal potassium levels (hyper- or hypokalemia) are associated with cardiac dysrhythmias which can be fatal [2,6]. For this reason, careful evaluation of the current electrolyte levels is imperative. Assessment of the sodium and ionized calcium levels should also be done at this time. In addition, it is not uncommon for the CRF patient to have an underlying acid/base imbalance due to the impeded ability to manage H^+ ions. This information is most useful in developing the plan for myocardial protection, prevention of electrolyte imbalances, and the stabilization of the acid/base balance in the immediate postoperative period. Careful intraoperative management may help avoid early dialysis.

While there are CRF patients who produce urine, diuresis is not a reliable means of managing fluid or electrolyte problems for these patients. Questions relating to current renal function such as the blood urea nitrogen and creatinine levels, as well as the hemoglobin and hematocrit, are all helpful in determining the need for intraoperative hemodialysis or ultrafiltration. A careful preoperative evaluation is the beginning of a successful intraoperative management plan that will help avoid postoperative complications related to the management of fluid and electrolyte issues in the CRF patient.

Intraoperative management

As previously noted, careful communication between the surgeon, anesthesiologist, and the perfusionist is critical to successful intraoperative management. Equally important is the realization that the intraoperative management plan will have a significant effect on the postoperative management and ultimate outcome for these patients with CRF.

Fluid management

The goal of fluid management during CPB is to maintain balance of a normovolemic state while also optimizing the hydrostatic and colloidal (osmotic) pressures within the intravascular space. Some of the variables impacting fluid management are as follows: the prime solution selected, the type of CPB circuit used (open or closed), the baseline blood volume, type/amount of cardioplegia solution, and preoperative hematocrit.

The selection of the priming solution for the CPB circuit in the CRF patient can be equated to pouring the foundation for a building. It is a crucial part of the management plan, as it establishes the base for future fluid management decisions. Initial calculations of the circulating blood volume and red cell mass are also important in this process. Utilizing the patient's weight, sex, and body structure, an estimate can be made (Table 1). The estimated blood volume, in milliliters, is the product of the patient's weight in kilograms (kg) multiplied by the X factor associated with their particular body type. Various crystalloid solutions such as 0.9 normal saline, lactated ringers, 5% dextrose, and electrolyte balanced (plasmalyte/normosol)

Table 1 Calculating estimated blood volumes (EBV).

Body type	"X" Male mL/kg	"X" Female mL/kg
Obese	60	55
Normal	65	60
Thin	70	65
Muscular	75	70

EBV = Wt. (kg) × X; resulting calculation in milliliter (mL).
Calculating red cell mass (RCM): RCM = EBV × HCT.

solutions have all been used to prime the CPB circuit [2,5–7]. In the ideal setting, completely isotonic priming solutions would be used. Some clinicians report using packed red blood cells, whole blood, and even fresh frozen plasma in their CPB prime [8]. But, in most cases the bypass circuit is primed with one of the previously noted crystalloid solutions.

It is beneficial to the patient to be able to remove the crystalloid prime in the circuit prior to the initiation of CPB while maintaining adequate hemodilution. If a cardioplegia system with a bridge for delivering blood alone is incorporated into the CPB circuit, it is a relatively safe and easy procedure to remove the crystalloid prime without the use of donated blood products. This is achieved by forcing the prime out of the circuit into an empty sterile intravenous bag via the cardioplegia bridge, while slowly draining the patient's blood into the venous reservoir just prior to commencing partial CPB [9]. Excellent communication between the surgeon, anesthesiologist, and perfusionist is required to prevent hypotension during this process.

The choice between an open (hard shell reservoir) or closed (soft or bag reservoir) CPB circuit has a large influence on the amount of additional volume administered during the time on CPB. Restricting the volume of fluid added during this period is crucial and has a direct impact on the overall operative outcome [10]. By utilizing a closed circuit the need for additional volume in order to maintain adequate flow is minimized. The inherent advantage to using a closed system is that it permits perfusion at normal calculated flow rates with a lower reservoir volume than an open system. For safety reasons regarding air transport via the arterial return line, an open system (hard shell reservoir) requires higher levels of volume in the venous reservoir. Some programs prefer the open system mainly due to decreased costs and ease of conversion to vacuum-assisted drainage. However, minimizing the addition of crystalloid fluids during the time on CPB by using a closed system will reduce the amount of fluid shifted to the interstitial spaces.

The intraoperative use of ultrafiltration is very useful in the removal of free water. Ultrafiltration uses hydrostatic pressure across a semipermeable membrane to facilitate the concentration of circulating blood volume. Postoperative complications from fluid overload such as pulmonary edema, impaired hemostasis, lowered hematocrit, and circulating mediators of the systemic inflammatory response can be mitigated through the judicious administration of fluids and the liberal use of ultrafiltration [11–14]. Darup and colleagues were the first to describe the use of ultrafiltration in conjunction with CPB in 1979 [15]. With improvements in filter designs and construction processes, using ultrafiltration parallel to CPB has become a standard of practice for the CRF patient.

Bridging the ultrafiltration blood path from the recirculation line on the CPB circuit to the cardiotomy reservoir provides flexibility in its utilization [9]. Ultrafiltration in parallel with the CPB circuit flow alleviates the need for a separate dedicated pump head. This configuration also allows for use of the hemoconcentrator for concentration of the remaining blood volume in the circuit at the termination of bypass, in a modified ultrafiltration setup.

Electrolyte management

While the goal of electrolyte management is to maintain all electrolytes within normal parameters, potassium deserves most of the attention. Life-threatening dysrhythmias are directly related to elevated or reduced levels of potassium. Hyperkalemia during the perioperative period has multiple sources, which include the following: decreased or absent potassium excretion, type of crystalloid solution used for priming, cardioplegia solution, hemolysis/blood trauma, infused blood products, drugs (i.e., succinylcholine) and acid/base balance management. The management of potassium has two distinct phases: (1) minimizing of potassium loading and (2) facilitating removal of excessive amounts of potassium.

As previously noted, electrolyte balanced solutions (plasmalyte, normosol), lactated ringers, and 0.9 normal saline have all been reported as priming solutions for CPB. When choosing a priming solution some issues to consider include: What are the current electrolyte levels? What is the patient's current state of intravascular volume? What is the current hematocrit? And how much crystalloid will be needed to achieve adequate hemodilution? Added effort should be made to remove the crystalloid prime prior to the initiation of CPB as described in the section on fluid management. Currently at our center, we prime the CPB circuit with 2 L of plasmalyte for deairing and then perform antegrade and retrograde autologous blood priming of the pump to reduce the total prime volume in the circuit to approximately 500 cm^3. Transfusions of donated blood products are often required due to the associated chronic anemia. In the cases where packed red blood cells are needed, every effort should be made to insure that they are washed prior to their infusion to remove any excess potassium.

Acid/base balance plays a key role in electrolyte management. Whether utilizing Ph stat or Alpha stat as your blood gas management technique, the pH, PaCO$_2$, and PaO$_2$ should be maintained within normal parameters. The importance can be demonstrated with the following example: a shift in the oxyhemoglobin dissociation curve to the left from a respiratory alkalosis impairs oxygen delivery at the tissue level. This impaired delivery will result in a metabolic acidosis causing the shifting of potassium out of the cells as a compensatory mechanism [16,20].

Myocardial protection utilizing a cold blood cardioplegia solution remains the standard of practice. Using a technique which allows for the delivery of high and low potassium containing solution, as well as blood alone, should provide sufficient flexibility to keep the heart cold and maintain an isoelectric state while minimizing the associated potassium load. Our technique consists of an initial dose of antegrade cold blood cardioplegia with a 2:1 ratio of blood to crystalloid cardioplegia with a high potassium component. Once an isoelectric state has been achieved, the cardioplegia solution is switched to blood alone to maintain the myocardial temperature between 10 and 15°C. Additional low-dose potassium cardioplegia is delivered to maintain an isoelectric state. In most cases, 200–300 cm^3 in the initial dose of potassium-rich cardioplegia solution is all that is needed to maintain the isoelectric state for the duration of the procedure. Some institutions employ a technique to scavenge the administered cardioplegia solution returning from the cardiotomy suction in order to avoid excessive potassium administration [21].

The hemoconcentrator or ultrafiltration filter can be used to remove excessive amounts of potassium. The sieving coefficient in most ultrafiltrators is 1.0 [22]. A solute whose sieving coefficient is 1.0 freely diffuses across a semipermeable membrane. While potassium freely diffuses across the membrane of the hemoconcentrator, it is necessary to add 0.9 normal saline to the perfusate in equal amounts to facilitate an adequate reduction in the potassium level, while maintaining the intravascular volume and hematocrit. After terminating CPB, the hemoconcentrator can be used to remove not only noncellular water, but also potassium from the blood that remains in the CPB circuit. This process results in the remaining blood for transfusion post bypass to have a high hematocrit and a low potassium level, similar to cell-saver salvaged blood, but retaining the plasma component.

The administration of calcium chloride, sodium bicarbonate, insulin, and 50% dextrose can be used to manipulate the extracellular potassium levels by forcing it into the intracellular space. This is a temporary solution and can result in problems controlling the potassium levels in the immediate postoperative period. Thus the patient receives a greater benefit by minimizing the administration of potassium and utilizing perioperative ultrafiltration to manage the potassium levels.

Flow rates and perfusion pressure

Normally, an adequate urine output (50–100 cm^3/h) is one of the parameters monitored in evaluating the adequacy of perfusion. This method is not possible in CRF patients undergoing cardiac surgery since they have little to no urine output. To maintain adequate flow and perfusion, it is recommended that the CPB flow rate is between 1.8 and 2.5 L/min/m^2 during periods of moderate hypothermia (25–28°C) [11,13]. Some institutions recommend monitoring of the venous saturation (VO$_2$) and maintaining it greater than 60% [2] while on bypass. Although frequently helpful, VO$_2$ measured in the venous line is not always representative of the actual O$_2$ delivery at the tissue level and may be less accurate in CRF patients. Most patients with CRF have AV fistulas that have demonstrated the potential for significant peripheral shunting [11]. The level of anticoagulation, the type, size, and location of the shunt, age of the implanted graft, and graft patency all affect the flow through the AV fistula [12]. In order to prevent regional ischemia from occurring, flow rates greater than 2.5 L/min/m^2 may be necessary to maintain adequate perfusion.

It is important to maintain an adequate perfusion pressure to keep the capillary beds open. But at the same time an excessively high mean perfusion pressure will result in a fluid shift into the interstitial spaces, creating an intravascular fluid deficit. The mean perfusion pressure should ideally be maintained between 50 mm Hg [11] and 65 mm Hg [13,19].

Intraoperative hemodialysis

Occasionally, it may be necessary to perform intraoperative hemodialysis for hyperkalemia. There is some evidence that the addition of hemodialysis to the perfusion circuit can decrease the morbidity and mortality of patients presenting with creatinine values greater than 2.5 mg/dL [24].

Some considerations for the intraoperative use of dialysis include the following: when to initiate the treatment, where to incorporate it into the CPB circuit, and type of dialysate to use. The time for initiation and duration of dialysis is dependent upon intravascular blood volume, electrolyte levels, and expected duration of CPB. Using the various access points on the CPB circuit is preferable to the patients A/V shunt. While the use of lactated ringers and peritoneal dialysis solution has been reported, the use of a sterile bicarbonate dialysate is shown to be beneficial in reducing potassium levels while maintaining normal glucose levels [25].

Special considerations

Arterial and venous cannulas for connecting the patient to the CPB circuit are usually based on the surgeon's preference. With advances in technology, cannula design and the resulting hemodynamic characteristics should not limit venous return or arterial inflow. Due to the diffuse atherosclerosis as part of the CRF process, these patients are at increased risk for stroke. The Embol-X arterial cannula, a relatively new arterial cannula with an intraarterial filter, may have some benefit in this patient population. Previous studies have documented capturing particulate emboli in greater than 90% of cases when the filter was deployed [26,27]. Although promising and somewhat intuitive, additional work needs to be done to document a clinically significant reduction in neurocognitive events with its routine use.

Most programs use some pharmacologic adjunct to reduce the systemic inflammatory response syndrome from CPB. Because the CRF patient is at increased risk for postoperative bleeding secondary to anemia, elevated BUN, platelet dysfunction, and poor nutrition, Trasylol (Bayer Pharmaceuticals Corporation, West Haven, CT) is frequently used. Trasylol has been shown to reduce the transfusion requirements in CRF patients undergoing cardiac surgery [28]. The dosing of Trasylol in these patients remains an issue. Trasylol is filtered by the glomeruli and physiologically handled by the kidneys similar to other small proteins. O'Connor and colleagues in a small group of patients with CRF noted that the terminal elimination half-life was significantly prolonged [29]. This has led several authors to suggest that the dose may need to be adjusted in patients with CRF [28,29]. Whether using regimen A (kallikrein-inhibiting) or regimen B (plasmin-inhibiting) when administering Trasylol, consideration should be given to adjusting the dose. Additional work involving larger numbers of patients is necessary to determine the most appropriate dose and its efficacy in this group of patients.

Discussion

Because these patients have diffuse atherosclerosis which frequently involves the ascending aorta, performing coronary artery bypass grafting off-pump seems to be an attractive option. However, due to the same disease process they tend to have diffuse coronary artery disease which may make accurate and complete revascularization difficult. A recent report by Dewey and colleagues comparing coronary artery bypass grafting in CRF patients showed improved long-term survival in those patients done on bypass [30].

The disease process associated with chronic renal dysfunction predisposes patients to accelerated cardiovascular disease frequently requiring surgical intervention. Currently, cardiac surgery in patients with CRF is best performed utilizing CPB to support the patient and facilitate the procedure. Careful planning preoperatively and special management intraoperatively are required by the cardiac surgical team to minimize the risk to the CRF patient. Timing of preoperative dialysis and the use of intraoperative ultrafiltration and hemodialysis have both been shown to decrease operative risk [23–25]. Patients with chronic renal dysfunction can safely undergo cardiac surgery with the use of CPB.

References

1 Lansing AM, Leb DE, Berman LB. Cardiovascular surgery in end stage renal failure. *JAMA* 1968; **204**:134–138.

2 Ko W, Kreiger KH, Isom OW. Cardiopulmonary bypass in dialysis patients. *Ann Thorac Surg* 1993; **55**(3):677–684.

3 Love JW, *et al*. Myocardial revascularization in patients with chronic renal failure. *J Thorac Cardiovasc Surg* 1980;**79**:625–627.

4 Murkin JM, Murphy DA, Finlayson DC, Walter JL. Hemodialysis during cardiopulmonary bypass: report of 12 cases. *Anesth Analg* 1987;**66**:899–901.

5 Zauder L, II. Anesthesia for patients who have terminal renal disease. *ASA Refresher Courses Anesthesiol* 1976;**4**:163–173.

6 Manhas DR, Merendino KA. The management of cardiac surgery in patients with chronic renal failure. *J Thorac Cardiovasc Surg* 1972;**63**(2):235–239.

7 Crawford FA, Jr, Selby JH, Jr, Bower JD, Lehan PH. Coronary revascularization in patients maintained on chronic hemodialysis. *Circulation* 1977 Oct;**56**(4 Pt 1):684–687.

8 Lambertti JJ, Cohn LH, Collins JJ, Jr. Cardiac surgery in patients undergoing renal dialysis or transplantation. *Ann Thorac Surg* 1975;**19**(2):135–141.

9 Sobieski MA, II, Slaughter MS, Hart D, Pappas PS, Tatooles AJ. Prospective study on cardiopulmonary bypass prime reduction and its effect on intraoperative blood product and hemoconcentrator use. *Perfusion* 2005;**20**:31–37.

10 Kubota T, Miyata A, Maeda A, Hirta K, Koizumi S, Ohba H. Continuous haemodi-afiltration during and after cardiopulmonary in renal patients. *Can J Anaesth* 1997;**44**(11):1182–1186.

11 Peper WA, Taylor PC, Paganinini EP, Svensson LG, Ghattas MA, Loop FD. Mortality and results after cardiac surgery in patients with end-stage renal disease. *Cleve Clin J Med* 1988;**55**(1):63–67.

12 Durmaz I, Buket S, Atay Y, *et al.* Cardiac surgery with cardiopulmonary bypass in patients with chronic renal failure. *J Thorac Cardiovasc Surg* 1999;**118**(2):306–315.

13 Allen FB, Kane PB. Anaesthesia for open-heart surgery in haemodialysis-dependent patients: a report of two cases. *Can Anaesth Soc J* 1982;**29**(2):158–162.

14 Rodriguez Moran M, Rodrigues JM, Ramos Boyero M, *et al.* Flow of dialysis fis-tulas. Noninvasive study performed with standard Doppler equipment. *Nephron* 1985;**40**:63–66.

15 Darup J, Bleese N, Kalmer P, *et al.* Hemofiltration during extracorporeal circulation. *Thorac Cardiovasc Surg* 1979;**27**:227–230.

16 Hakim M, Wheeldon D, Bethune DW, Milstein BB, English TA, Wallwork J. Haemodialysis and haemofiltration on cardiopulmonary bypass. *Thorax* 1985;**40** (2):101–106.

17 Karzai W, Priebe HJ. Oxygen consumption in hemodialysis patients undergoing cardiopulmonary bypass. *J Cardiothorac Vasc Anesth* 1998;**12**(4):415–417.

18 Sutton RG. Renal considerations, dialysis, and ultrafiltration during cardiopul-monary bypass [review]. *Int Anesthesiol Clin.* 1996;**34**(2):165–176.

19 Journois D, Pouard P, Greely W, *et al.* Hemofiltration during cardiopulmonary by-pass in pediatric cardiac surgery: effects on hemostasis, cytokines, and complement components. *Anesthesiology* 1994;**81**:1181–1189.

20 Andreasson S, Gothberg S, Berggren H, *et al.* Hemofiltration modifies complement activation after extracorporeal circulation in infants. *Ann Thorac Surg* 1993;**56**:1515–1517.

21 Ashraf SS, Shaukat N, Kamaly ID, Durri A, Doran B, Grotte GJ. Determinants of early and late mortality in patients with end-stage renal disease undergoing cardiac surgery. *Scand J Thorac Cardiovasc Surg* 1995;**29**(4):187–193.

22 Williams JS, Crawford FA, Jr, Kratz JM, Riley JB. Cardiac surgery for patients main-tained on chronic hemodialysis. *J S C Med Assoc* 1991;**87**(12):569–573.

23 Sutton RG. Renal considerations, dialysis, and ultrafiltration during cardiopul-monary bypass. *Int Anesthesiol Clin* 1996;**34**(2):165–176.

24 Durmaz I, Yagdi T, Calkavur T, *et al.* Prophylactic dialysis in patients with renal dysfunction undergoing on-pump coronary artery bypass surgery. *Ann Thorac Surg* 2003;**75**(3):859–864.

25 Tobe SW, Murphy PM, Goldberg P, *et al.* A new sterile bicarbonate dialysis solution for use during cardiopulmonary bypass. *ASAIO J* 1999;**45**(3):157–159.

26 Banbury MK, Kouchoukos NT, Allen KB, *et al.* ICEM 2000 Investigators. Emboli cap-ture using the Embol-X intra-aortic filter in cardiac surgery: a multi-centered ran-domized trial of 1,289 patients. *Ann Thorac Surg* 2003;**76**(2):508–515; discussion 515.

27 Sobieski M, Pappas PS, Tatooles AJ, Slaughter MS. Embol-X Intra-aortic filtration system: capturing particulate emboli in the cardiac surgery patient. *J Extra Corpor Technol* 2005;**37**:222–226.

28 Lemmer JH, Metzdorff MT, Krause AH, *et al*. Aprotinin use in patients with dialysis-dependent renal failure undergoing cardiac operations. *J Thorac Cardiovasc Surg* 1996: **112**:192–194.

29 O'Connor CJ, Brown DV, Avramov M, Barnes S, O'Connor HN, Tuman KJ. The impact of renal dysfunction on aprotinin pharmacokinetics during cardiopulmonary bypass. *Anesth Analg* 1999;**89**:1101–1107.

30 Dewey TM, Herbert MA, Prince SL, *et al*. Does coronary artery bypass graft surgery improve survival among patients with end-stage renal disease? *Ann Thorac Surg* 2006;**81**:591–598.

CHAPTER 4

Coronary artery bypass grafting in dialysis-dependent renal failure patients

Matthew Forrester, William Cohn

Introduction

Cardiovascular disease is the leading cause of morbidity and mortality among patients with renal failure [1], accounting for 44% of all-cause mortality [2]. Of these deaths, approximately 22% are due to acute myocardial infarction (AMI) [2]. Overall mortality after AMI for patients receiving long-term dialysis is 59.3% at 1 year and 89.9% at 5 years; mortality in these patients from all cardiac causes is about 40% at 1 year and 70% at 5 years [3]. Dialysis-dependent renal failure (DDRF) patients frequently have multiple comorbidities in addition to cardiovascular disease [4]. As of 2000, approximately 281,000 patients in the United States were undergoing dialysis treatment, and it is estimated that as many as 520,000 patients will require dialysis by 2010 [2]. Furthermore, patients >65 years often require more frequent dialysis [5]. Among DDRF patients >65 years, cardiac disease accounts for 131.1 deaths per 1000 patients compared to 85.3 deaths per 1000 patients for dialysis patients between 20 and 64 years old [6].

Thus, effective treatment of cardiovascular disease in these patients could potentially improve both functional status and survival. For example, in end-stage renal patients, coronary revascularization may improve outcomes after kidney transplantation [7]. Although the optimal approach to revascularization—percutaneous coronary intervention (PCI) or coronary artery bypass grafting (CABG)—remains a subject of controversy [3,8–16], the increased incidence of cardiovascular disease and the increasing number of patients requiring dialysis necessitate our investigating the best approach for treating coronary artery disease in this patient population.

Coronary artery bypass grafting in dialysis-dependent patients

The significant comorbidities present in DDRF patients undergoing CABG lead to higher morbidity and mortality rates compared to those of all patients who undergo CABG procedures [17,18]. After CABG procedures, DDRF patients have poor short- and long-term survival [4,8,18,19] and a high incidence of postoperative stroke [17,18,20,21], infection [19], bleeding [12,18,22,23], and cardiac complications [17]. They also require prolonged mechanical ventilation [14,18,19,21,24] and longer postoperative stays [22,24]. The comorbidities commonly present with renal failure, such as diabetes, recent myocardial infarction, low ejection fraction, increased age, chronic pulmonary disease, and cerebrovascular disease, are shown to be independent predictors of postoperative mortality after CABG [25]. Liu *et al.* [17] (Northern New England Cardiovascular Disease Study Group) report that in a prospective cohort study of 15,500 patients undergoing CABG between 1992 and 1997 preoperative dialysis dependence is a strong independent predictor for in-hospital mortality. Although DDRF patients had more severe coronary disease with more comorbidities than did non-dialysis patients, multivariate analysis revealed that DDRF patients were 3.1 times more likely to die in the hospital after a CABG procedure. Significantly higher postoperative stroke and mediastinitis rates (4.3 and 3.6% vs 1.7 and 1.2%, respectively) were also observed [17].

Franga *et al.* [18] used the Society of Thoracic Surgeons database to compare patients undergoing CABG, regardless of renal function, and found that DDRF patients had a higher incidence of mortality (11.4% vs 2.8%), cerebrovascular accident (7% vs 1.7%), and cardiac arrest (7% vs 1.5%) in the early postoperative period. The overall complication rate in the early postoperative period was also substantially greater in these patients (73% vs 32%) [18]. Despite the increased risk associated with surgery in DDRF patients, several reports have demonstrated acceptable morbidity and mortality rates and an improved quality of life [12,14,16,26,27]. Coronary revascularization in DDRF patients has been investigated since 1974, when Menzoin *et al.* [28] reported the first coronary bypass procedure in a patient with chronic renal failure. Until recently, however, most studies have been limited to small retrospective analyses of data from single-institution experiences, making it difficult to draw conclusions. Data from large multivariate studies are needed to identify the best clinical practices which result in improved outcomes. Table 1 demonstrates the increased, yet variable, operative mortality from several authors.

A prospective analysis of 15,500 patients by Dacey *et al.* [4] (Northern New England Cardiovascular Disease Study Group) revealed crude

Table 1 Patient populations and in-hospital mortality rates in recent series.

Reference	Number of patients	In-hospital mortality*
Herzog (1999) [29]	7419	12.5%
Labrousse (1999) [7]	82	14.6%
Agirbasli (2000) [8]	130	6.9%
Liu (2000) [17]	279	12.2%
Khaitan (2000) [19]	70	14.3%
Franga (2000) [18]	44	11.4%
Nishida (2001) [30]	105	4.8%[†]
Dacey (2002) [4]	283	12.1%
Herzog (2002) [9]	6668	8.6%
Gelsomino (2002) [31]	28	7.1%

*In-hospital mortality defined as 30-day mortality.
[†]Total in-hospital mortality was 12.4% when patients who died beyond 30 days after CABG but before discharge are included.

in-hospital mortality rates of 12.1% for DDRF patients compared to 3.0% for nonrenal failure patients; 5-year mortality was 44.2 and 16.5%, respectively [4]. These results are consistent with other results of studies conducted after 1990, which have shown a combined in-hospital mortality of 12% [5,7,8,10,12,15,16,18,19,23,26,27,30]. Long-term results are difficult to compare given the widely varied follow-up, but reported actuarial survivals range from 55 to 70% at 3 years [7,12,23,26] and from 32 to 69% at 5 years [5,7,9,18,27,30].

In general, DDRF patients have higher baseline rates of diabetes, peripheral vascular disease (PVD), and chronic obstructive pulmonary disease; lower ejection fractions and higher left ventricular end-diastolic pressures; a higher incidence of left main disease; and more diseased vessels. DDRF patients are also more likely to have a history of congestive heart failure (CHF), myocardial infarction, and unstable angina at baseline compared to nondialysis patients [4,17]. Stratified analysis showed that the annual death rate among patients with renal failure alone was twice that of non-renal failure patients; the death rate among those with renal failure and diabetes or PVD was more than six times that of nonrenal failure patients. The 5-year mortality associated with CABG was 21.5% in patients with renal failure alone and 57.8% in patients with renal failure and diabetes or PVD. Although the presence of preoperative DDRF was a highly significant predictor of decreased long-term survival in the northern New England study, mortality rates were similar to the generally acceptable rates of previous studies. However, there is much room for improvement.

Coronary artery bypass grafting versus percutaneous coronary intervention

Although acceptable morbidity and mortality rates and improved quality of life have been demonstrated after CABG in DDRF patients, whether surgical revascularization is superior to percutaneous revascularization remains a subject of debate.

Using data from the U.S. Renal Data System (USRDS) database for a retrospective review of 14,000 dialysis patients who underwent either CABG or percutaneous transluminal coronary angioplasty (PTCA) between 1978 and 1995, Herzog et al. [29] report that despite a higher in-hospital mortality rate for CABG, long-term survival was more favorable for the surgical patients. Overall in-hospital mortality was 12.5% for CABG and 5.4% for PTCA, but the 1-year, all-cause mortality was 29.4% after CABG and 31.1% after PTCA. Unadjusted long-term survival differences between the two groups were not drastic. Unadjusted 2-year, event-free survival for all-cause and cardiac death was 56.9 and 75.8% after CABG and 52.9 and 72.5% after PTCA, respectively. However, after adjusting for demographics, comorbidity, and time frame of revascularization, the survival improvement for CABG over PTCA was 9% for all-cause death, 15% for cardiac death, 63% for AMI alone, and 31% for AMI and cardiac death combined.

Analysis of independent predictors of all-cause death, cardiac death, and AMI was performed for both groups. Old age (≥75 years) and diabetes were the most powerful predictors of all-cause death and cardiac death for all patients undergoing revascularization. Most comorbid conditions were also significant predictors of all-cause and cardiac death. The risk of AMI increased 21% in patients with diabetic renal failure and significantly increased in patients with atherosclerotic heart disease and CHF. However, the most powerful predictor of postoperative AMI was the method of revascularization: CABG resulted in a significantly lower rate. Although this study revealed a multitude of differential effects of PTCA and CABG, the USRDS database used in the study fails to provide important clinical prognostic factors, such as left ventricular function and severity of CAD. Moreover, the study does not take into account improvements in PCI, particularly the use of stents. It does, however, provide substantial evidence that, despite higher periprocedural mortality, CABG provides better long-term results for dialysis patients.

In a more recent retrospective analysis of nearly 16,000 patients, again using data from the USRDS database, Herzog et al. [9] compared results of CABG, PTCA, and coronary stenting among dialysis patients. The 2-year survival was 56.4, 48.2, and 48.4% after CABG, PTCA, and stenting, respectively. After adjusting for comorbidities, the relative risk (RR) for CABG was 0.80 for all-cause death and 0.72 for cardiac death. However, once again, the CABG patients had a higher in-hospital mortality than did the PTCA and stent patients (8.6% vs 6.4% and 4.1%) [9].

In the largest single-institution analysis, Agirbasli *et al.* [8] report their 10-year experience with CABG and PTCA in DDRF patients. Again, higher in-hospital mortality was observed for CABG patients (6.9%) than for PTCA patients (1.6%). In this study, however, there was no significant difference in 1-year mortality for CABG and PTCA (27 and 25%). PTCA was performed more often in patients with early CAD, but CABG was usually performed in patients with more advanced disease (e.g., 3-vessel or left main disease); thus, selection bias may have affected the results. There was also significant interaction between the type of revascularization and the number of diseased vessels. PTCA was associated with a lower mortality in patients with 2-vessel disease and a higher mortality in those with left main disease, which suggests that PTCA may be an appropriate treatment for a select group of DDRF patients. However, the need for repeat revascularization (i.e., PTCA) was also significantly higher in the PTCA group (16%) than in the CABG group (2.1%). After 1 year, 7.5% of the PTCA patients had to undergo CABG while none of the CABG patients had to undergo a repeat CABG procedure [8].

Such studies demonstrate an overall survival advantage for DDRF patients who undergo CABG. However, treatment may be influenced by preoperative comorbid conditions such as severity of CAD and degree of left ventricular dysfunction [11]. In a retrospective study comparing 59,600 patients undergoing isolated CABG or PCI, Szczech *et al.* [11] investigated comparative survival while controlling for confounding factors, including severity of renal dysfunction and degree of CAD and left ventricular dysfunction. As demonstrated in previous studies [4,17], dialysis-dependent patients had poorer left ventricular function and more severe CAD than did patients with mild or no renal dysfunction. In this study, a greater proportion of dialysis patients had diabetes mellitus, PVD, cerebrovascular disease, left ventricular hypertrophy, chronic obstructive pulmonary disease, and CHF. Further, patients undergoing CABG had poorer left ventricular function, more severe CAD, and greater frequency of comorbidities than did those undergoing PCI. Independent predictors of mortality included increasing severity of CAD, increasing age, an ejection fraction <30%, a history of stroke, PVD, and persistent ventricular arrhythmia. Adjusted survival at 1, 2, and 3 years was 84.1, 77.4, and 65.9% for CABG patients and 70.8, 51.9, and 46.1% for PCI patients, respectively. In patients with mild or no renal dysfunction, there was no demonstrated survival benefit associated with CABG [32].

Despite the higher periprocedural mortality rates associated with CABG in dialysis patients [8,9,29], most studies report better long-term survival after CABG than after PCI [8–11,29,32,33]. In the aforementioned studies, in-hospital mortality ranged from 6.9 to 12.5% for CABG and from 1.6 to 5.7% for PCI, 1-year mortality from 15.9 to 29.4% for CABG and from 25 to 29.7% for PCI, and 2-year mortality from 22.6 to 43.6% for CABG and from 48.1 to 59.6% for PCI [8,9,11,29]. In addition, several studies have demonstrated an unacceptably high rate of restenosis [10,13,34–36] and the increased occurrence of cardiac events [34,35] after PCI in this subset of patients. Thus, surgical revascularization is generally accepted as the preferred treatment for CAD in dialysis-dependent patients, despite the higher periprocedural mortality rate.

Surgical technique

Although CABG has been shown to improve survival and quality of life, there remain substantially higher morbidity and mortality rates among DDRF patients as compared to patients with mild or no renal dysfunction. Presently, there is debate regarding the optimal surgical technique for CABG in DDRF patients. Some investigators have suggested that use of more arterial grafts may improve results and others have investigated the detrimental affects of cardiopulmonary bypass (CPB) in this patient population.

Although there is a higher rate of AMI and cardiac death in DDRF patients who undergo CABG than there is in nonrenal failure patients, repeat revascularization rates are drastically lower in surgical patients than in PCI patients. In the largest-reported single-institution experience, Agirbasli *et al.* [8] report that at 1-year follow-up, 2.1% of CABG patients required PTCA, significantly lower than the 16% of PTCA patients who required a repeat PTCA procedure. In the same period, 2.9% of CABG patients had an AMI compared to 4.7% of PTCA patients [8]. In a sample of 105 chronic dialysis patients undergoing CABG in Japan, 6 patients had myocardial infarctions, 13 required PTCA, and 1 required redo CABG during long-term follow-up, yielding a revascularization rate of 13% [30]. In contrast, the Bypass Angioplasty Revascularization Investigation (BARI) investigators found that, regardless of renal function, 8% of patients who underwent CABG required additional revascularization in the first 5 years after surgery [37].

Use of arterial conduits may reduce graft occlusion and improve long-term patency [10]. Thus, arterial grafts have been used in high-risk patients in an attempt to reduce postoperative complications and improve long-term results [38]. Labrousse *et al.* [7] found that use of the internal mammary artery (IMA) as an arterial conduit was directly related to lower hospital mortality. Additionally, because of the greater incidence of vascular disease in DDRF patients, atherosclerosis of the ascending aorta is a concern during heart surgery. Surgical manipulation during cannulation, cross-clamping, or proximal vein graft anastomoses is a potentially dangerous source of systemic emboli [39]. When severe calcification of the ascending aorta is suspected, use of arterial conduits avoids aortic anastomoses and, thus, reduces the risk of neurologic events.

However, it has been suggested that chronic hemodialysis may pose problems for use of IMA bypass grafts. Because chronic hemodialysis patients often undergo treatment via an upper-extremity arteriovenous fistula, a steal phenomenon may occur; whereby hemodialysis reduces flow to the IMA ipsilateral to the arteriovenous fistula [40–42]. Clinical observation of angina episodes during hemodialysis in patients with patent IMA bypass grafts has prompted investigation into this phenomenon. Gaudino *et al.* [40] studied 5 patients requiring chronic hemodialysis treatment via a left upper-extremity arteriovenous fistula who had undergone left IMA to left anterior descending (LAD) bypass grafting. With the dialysis pump off, echocardiography showed a local reduction in vascular resistance at the fistula site that was transmitted to the ipsilateral IMA, evidenced by an increase in end-diastolic volume (EDV) and time-averaged mean velocity (TAMV) and a consequent reduction in the pulsatility index (PI). With the dialysis pump on, flow through the fistula increased as expected, and flow in the ipsilateral IMA graft markedly decreased, with a reduced peak systolic velocity (PSV), EDV, and TAMV and an increased PI. Conversely, there was no substantial hemodynamic effect observed in the contralateral IMA. Increased pump flow rates led to more drastic changes in flow. Moreover, in each case, reduction of IMA flow led to concomitant hypokinesia of the anterior left ventricular wall, which resolved when the dialysis pump was turned off. Three of the five patients also reported symptoms of referred myocardial ischemia. Thus, the report suggests that care should be taken to avoid use of the IMA ipsilateral to an arteriovenous fistula.

Similarly, off-pump coronary artery bypass (OP-CAB) is increasingly being performed in high-risk patients in an attempt to improve results [43–45]. Use of CPB during heart surgery carries several inherent risks, including bleeding, altered hemoglobin concentrations, potential neuro-logic deficits, fluid and electrolyte imbalances, hemolysis, and systemic inflammatory responses [18,46]. In addition to oxygen-free radicals gen-erated by CPB, a number of inflammatory mediators are released during extracorporeal circulation, which may contribute to multiple organ dys-function [38,47]. Avoidance of CPB has been associated with decreased postoperative mortality, reduced incidence of perioperative arrhythmia, superior renal protection, and shorter hospital stays [44,45,48,49]. Given the already high comorbidity in DDRF patients, it has been suggested that OP-CAB may improve results in this population. In a retrospective review, Papadimitriou *et al.* [38] assessed the results of 19 patients who underwent CABG with the aid of CPB and 15 patients who underwent OP-CAB. There were no deaths in the CPB group and one sudden death in the OP-CAB group. However, early hemodialysis for hyperkalemia was required in 3 of 19 patients in the CPB group and in 1 of 15 patients in the OP-CAB group. Furthermore, in order to maintain the same blood urea nitrogen (BUN) target value, patients in the CPB group required 38% more dialysis postoperatively than did patients in the OP-CAB group, suggesting that the CPB group was more catabolic as a whole [38]. Additional experience with OP-CAB in the select group of patients is necessary to determine if avoiding the use of CPB support may improve the perioperative outcomes.

Revascularization in renal transplant recipients

Just like the DDRF patients, cardiovascular disease is the leading cause of death among renal transplant recipients. Since up to 50% of deaths af-ter renal transplant are due to cardiovascular events, it also represents a significant cause of organ loss [50]. Ischemic heart disease is one of the more common fatal cardiovascular events. Herzog and colleagues have recently demonstrated an improved survival in renal transplant patients that had an aggressive revascularization (CAB) compared to less aggres-sive modalities (PTCA) [51]. Interestingly, this improvement compared to PTCA was present whether an IMA was used or saphenous vein as the bypass conduit. Eschertzhuber has also demonstrated a decrease in post-transplant cardiac events in renal transplant recipients that had subsequent revascularization procedures [52]. In the renal transplant patient, there is concern due to the use of immunosuppressive drugs and the associated risk factors that led to renal failure and its effect on surgical complications. Frequently, clinicians are aware of the morbidity and mortality associated with surgical revascularization in DDRF and assume that it is similar in renal transplant recipients. Massad and colleagues have demonstrated a survival advantage in patients undergoing CAB with renal transplants compared to those with DDRF [53]. Overall, the morbidity and mortality in his series for renal transplant patients were similar to those patients undergoing CAB that had an elevated creatinine but were not on dialysis. As more aggressive evaluation of cardiovascular disease in renal transplant recipients is performed, additional knowledge will be gained as to the best method of revascularization in this subset of chronic renal failure patients.

Discussion

Ischemic heart disease is common in the chronic renal failure patient that is dialysis dependent. The need for dialysis is an independent predictor of morbidity and mortality in these patients who require coronary artery revascularization. Despite an increased early mortality for CAB compared to PCI, CAB appears to have improved long-term survival and the need for fewer repeat procedures. There is significant room for improvement in decreasing the early operative morbidity and mortality in DDRF patients. In most patients an IMA should be used but may require some consideration in patients that have a large ipsilateral fistula particularly if located in the upper arm. In addition, those DDRF patients who have gone on to renal transplantation appear to have a similar benefit of CAB over PCI for the treatment of ischemic heart disease. As the population ages and more people require dialysis for their chronic renal insufficiency, it is imperative that we continue to evaluate this high-risk population to determine the most successful and cost-effective mode of treatment for their ischemic heart disease.

References

1 U.S. Renal Data System. 1998 Annual Data Report. *Am J Kidney Dis* 1998:**32**(2, suppl. 1):S79–S90.
2 *USRDS 2000 Annual Data Report*. NIH Publication No. 00-3176. National Institutes of Health, Bethesda, MD; 2000:589–684;69–75.
3 Herzog CA, Ma JZ, Collins AJ. Poor long-term survival after acute myocardial infarction among patients on long-term dialysis. *N Engl J Med* 1998;**339**(12):799–805.
4 Dacey LJ, Liu JY, Braxton JH, *et al*. Northern New England Cardiovascular Disease Study Group. Long-term survival of dialysis patients after coronary bypass grafting. *Ann Thorac Surg* 2002;**74**(2):458–462; discussion 462–463.
5 Gelsomino S, Morocutti G, Masullo G, *et al*. Open heart surgery in patients with dialysis-dependent renal insufficiency. *J Card Surg* 2001;**16**(5):400–407.
6 *U.S. Renal Data System 1997*. Bethesda MD, National Institutes of Health; 1997.

7 Labrousse L, de Vincentiis C, Madonna F, Deville C, Roques X, Baudet E. Early and long term results of coronary artery bypass grafts in patients with dialysis dependent renal failure. Eur J Cardiothorac Surg 1999;**15**(5):691–696.

8 Agirbasli M, Weintraub WS, Chang GL, *et al.* Outcome of coronary revascularization in patients on renal dialysis. Am J Card 2000;**86**(4):395–399.

9 Herzog CA, Ma JZ, Collins AJ. Comparative survival of dialysis patients in the United States after coronary angioplasty, coronary artery stenting, and coronary artery bypass surgery and impact of diabetes. *Circulation* 2002;**106**(17):2207–2211.

10 Koyanagi T, Nishida H. Kitamura M, *et al.* Comparison of clinical outcomes of coronary artery bypass grafting and percutaneous transluminal coronary angioplasty in renal dialysis patients. *Ann Thorac Surg* 1996;**61**(6):1793–1796.

11 Szczech LA, Reddan DN, Owen WF, *et al.* Differential survival after coronary revascularization procedures among patients with renal insufficiency. *Kidney Int* 2001;**60**(1):292–299.

12 Batiuk TD, Kurtz SB, Oh JK, Orszulak TA. Coronary artery bypass operation in dialysis patients. *Mayo Clin Proc* 1991;**66**(1):45–53.

13 Rinehart AL, Herzog CA, Collins AJ, Flack JM, Ma JZ, Opsahl JA. A comparison of coronary angioplasty and coronary artery bypass grafting outcomes in chronic dialysis patients. *Am J Kidney Dis* 1995;**25**(2):281–290.

14 Deutsch E, Bernstein RC, Addonizio P, Kussmaul WG, III. Coronary artery bypass surgery in patients on chronic hemodialysis. A case-control study. *Ann Intern Med* 1989;**110**(5):369–372.

Deutsch E, Bernstein RC, Addonizio P, Kussmaul WG, III. Coronary artery bypass surgery in patients on chronic hemodialysis. A case-control study [erratum]. *Ann Intern Med* 1989;**110**(9):752.

15 Samuels LE, Sharma S, Morris RJ, *et al.* Coronary artery bypass grafting in patients with chronic renal failure: a reappraisal. *J Card Surg* 1996;**11**(2):128–133; discussion 134–135.

16 Owen CH, Cummings RG, Sell TL, Schwab SJ, Jones RH, Glower DD. Coronary artery bypass grafting in patients with dialysis-dependent renal failure. *Ann Thorac Surg* 1994;**58**(6):1729–1733.

17 Liu JY, Birkmeyer NJ, Sanders JH, *et al.* Risks of morbidity and mortality in dialysis patients undergoing coronary artery bypass surgery. Northern New England Cardiovascular Disease Study Group. *Circulation* 2000;**102**(24):2973–2977.

18 Franga DL, Kratz JM, Crumbley AJ, Zellner JL, Stroud MR, Crawford FA. Early and long-term results of coronary artery bypass grafting in dialysis patients. *Ann Thorac Surg* 2000;**70**(3):813–818; discussion 819.

19 Khaitan L, Sutter FP, Goldman SM. Coronary artery bypass grafting in patients who require long-term dialysis. *Ann Thorac Surg* 2000;**69**(4):1135–1139.

20 Kaul TK, Fields BL, Reddy MA, Kahn DR. Cardiac operations in patients with end-stage renal disease. *Ann Thorac Surg* 1994;**57**(3):691–696.

21 Christiansen S, Claus M, Philipp T, Reidemeister JC. Cardiac surgery in patients with end-stage renal failure. *Clin Nephrol.* 1997;**48**(4):246–252.

22 Wong D, Thompson G, Buth K, Sullivan J, Ali I. Angiographic coronary diffuseness and outcomes in dialysis patients undergoing coronary artery bypass grafting surgery. *Eur J Cardiothorac Surg* 2003;**24**(3):388–392.

23 Jahangiri M, Wright J, Edmondson S, Magee P. Coronary artery bypass graft surgery in dialysis patients. *Heart* 1997;**78**(4):343–345.

24 Hirose H, Amano A, Takahashi A. Efficacy of off-pump coronary artery bypass grafting for the patients on chronic hemodialysis. *Jpn J Thorac Cardiovasc Surg.* 2001;**49**(12):693–699.

25 Kurki TS, Kataja M. Preoperative prediction of postoperative morbidity in coronary artery bypass grafting. *Ann Thorac Surg* 1996;**61**(6):1740–1745.

26 Castelli P, Condemi AM, Munari M. Immediate and long-term results of coronary revascularization in patients undergoing chronic hemodialysis. *Eur J Cardiothorac Surg* 1999;**15**(1):51–54.

27 Blum U, Skupin M, Wagner R, Matheis G, Oppermann F, Satter P. Early and long-term results of cardiac surgery in dialysis patients. *Cardiovasc Surg* 1994;**2**(1):97–100.

28 Menzoin J, Davis RC, Idelson BA, *et al.* Coronary artery bypass surgery and renal transplantation: a case report. *Ann Surg* 1974;**179**:63–64.

29 Herzog CA, Ma JZ, Collins AJ. Long-term outcome of dialysis patients in the United States with coronary revascularization procedures. *Kidney Int* 1999;**56**(1):324–332.

30 Nishida H, Uchikawa S, Chikazawa G, *et al.* Coronary artery bypass grafting in 105 patients with hemodialysis-dependent renal failure. *Artif Organs* 2001;**25**(4):268–272.

31 Gelsomino S, Morocutti G, Masullo G, *et al.* Open heart surgery in patients with dialysis-dependent renal insufficiency. *J Cardiac Surg* 2001;**16**(5):400–407.

32 Reddan DN, Szczech LA, Tuttle RH, *et al.* Chronic kidney disease, mortality, and treatment strategies among patients with clinically significant coronary artery disease. *J Am Soc Nephrol* 2003;**14**(9):2373–2380.

33 Simsir SA, Kohlman-Trigoboff D, Flood R, Lindsay J, Smith BM. A comparison of coronary artery bypass grafting and percutaneous transluminal coronary angioplasty in patients on hemodialysis. *Cardiovasc Surg* 1998;**6**(5):500–505.

34 Schoebel FC, Gradaus F, Ivens K, *et al.* Restenosis after elective coronary balloon angioplasty in patients with end stage renal disease: a case-control study using quantitative coronary angiography. *Heart* 1997;**78**(4):337–342.

35 Marso SP, Gimple LW, Philbrick JT, DiMarco JP. Effectiveness of percutaneous coronary interventions to prevent recurrent coronary events in patients on chronic hemodialysis. *Am J Cardiol* 1998;**82**(3):378–380.

36 Kahn JK, Rutherford BD, McConahay DR, Johnson WL, Giorgi LV, Hartzler GO. Short- and long-term outcome of percutaneous transluminal coronary angioplasty in chronic dialysis patients. *Am Heart J* 1990;**119**(3 Pt 1):484–489.

37 Anonymous. Comparison of coronary bypass surgery with angioplasty in patients with multivessel disease. The Bypass Angioplasty Revascularization Investigation (BARI) Investigators. [erratum appears in N Engl J Med 1997 Jan 9;336(2):147]. *N Engl J Med* 1996;**335**(4):217–225.
Anonymous. Comparison of coronary bypass surgery with angioplasty in patients with multivessel disease. The Bypass Angioplasty Revascularization Investigation (BARI) Investigators [erratum]. *N Engl J Med* 1997;**336**(2):147.

38 Papadimitriou LJ, Marathias KP, Alivizatos PA, *et al.* Safety and efficacy of off-pump coronary artery bypass grafting in chronic dialysis patients. *Artif Organs* 2003;**27**(2):174–180.

39 Gaudino M, Glieca F, Alessandrini F, *et al.* The unclampable ascending aorta in coronary artery bypass patients: a surgical challenge of increasing frequency. *Circulation* 2000;**102**(13):1497–1502.

40 Gaudino M, Serricchio M, Luciani N, *et al.* Risks of using internal thoracic artery grafts in patients in chronic hemodialysis via upper extremity arteriovenous fistula. *Circulation*. 2003;**107**(21):2653–2655.

41 Kato H, Ikawa S, Hayashi A, Yokoyama K. Internal mammary artery steal in a dialysis patient. *Ann Thorac Surg* 2003;**75**(1):270–271.

42 Crowley SD, Butterly DW, Peter RH, Schwab SJ. Coronary steal from a left internal mammary artery coronary bypass graft by a left upper extremity arteriovenous hemodialysis fistula. *Am J Kidney Dis* 2002;**40**(4):852–855.

43 Akiyama K, Ogasawara K, Inoue T, *et al.* Myocardial revascularization without cardiopulmonary bypass in patients with operative risk factors. *Ann Thorac Cardiovasc Surg* 1999;**5**(1):31–35.

44 Yokoyama T, Baumgartner FJ, Gheissari A, Capouya ER, Panagiotides GP, Declusin RJ. Off-pump versus on-pump coronary bypass in high-risk subgroups. *Ann Thorac Surg* 2000;**70**(5):1546–1550.

45 Boyd WD, Desai ND, Del Rizzo DF, Novick RJ, McKenzie FN, Menkis AH. Off-pump surgery decreases postoperative complications and resource utilization in the elderly. *Ann Thorac Surg* 1999;**68**(4):1490–1493.

46 Horst M, Mehlhorn U, Hoerstrup SP, Suedkamp M, de Vivie ER. Cardiac surgery in patients with end-stage renal disease: 10-year experience. *Ann Thorac Surg* 2000;**69**(1):96–101.

47 Cremer J, Martin M, Redl H, *et al.* Systemic inflammatory response syndrome after cardiac operations. *Ann Thorac Surg* 1996;**61**(6):1714–1720.

48 Ascione R, Lloyd CT, Underwood MJ, Gomes WJ, Angelini GD. On-pump versus off-pump coronary revascularization: evaluation of renal function. *Ann Thorac Surg* 1999;**68**(2):493–498.

49 Arom KV, Flavin TF, Emery RW, Kshettry VR, Janey PA, Petersen RJ. Safety and efficacy of off-pump coronary artery bypass grafting. *Ann Thorac Surg* 2000;**69**(3):704–710.

50 Rigatto C. Management of cardiovascular disease in the renal transplant recipient. *Cardiol Clin* 2005;**23**:331–342.

51 Herzog CA, Ma JZ, Collins AJ. Long-term outcome of renal transplant recipients in the United States after coronary revascularization procedures. *Circulation* 2004;**109**:2866–2871.

52 Eschertzhuber S, Hohlrleder M, Boesmueller C, *et al.* Incidence of coronary heart disease and cardiac events in patients undergoing kidney and pancreatic transplantation. *Transplant Proc* 2005;**37**(2):1297–1300.

53 Massad MG, Kpodonu J, Lee J, *et al.* Outcome of coronary artery bypass operations in patients with renal insufficiency with and without renal transplantation. *Chest* 2005;**128**(2):855–862.

Surgical treatment of valvular heart disease in end-stage renal failure

Mark S. Slaughter

Introduction

Dialysis for end-stage renal disease (ESRD) was made widely available as a treatment option in 1972 when these patients were granted Medicare coverage. Currently, there are over 200,000 patients on dialysis in the United States and with the aging of the population it has been predicted that there will be 350,000 patients by 2010 [1]. Despite improvements in technology, techniques, and management of fluid and electrolyte abnormalities, dialysis as renal replacement therapy continues to have a significant impact on survival. The leading cause of death for this group of patients is cardiovascular disease as noted in the previous chapters. Although coronary artery disease is the leading cause of morbidity and mortality in this group, it has been estimated that approximately 30% [2] will develop calcific valvular heart disease. The surgical treatment of valvular heart disease in these dialysis-dependent patients continues to be associated with significant morbidity and mortality and warrants further investigation and review.

Etiology

Chronic renal failure results in alterations in electrolyte metabolism including phosphate and calcium. This abnormal calcium and phosphate metabolism in conjunction with hypertension has been associated with accelerated calcification of the aortic and mitral valves [3–7]). Interestingly, the abnormal calcification in the aortic valve tends to occur in the leaflets whereas in the mitral valve it occurs predominantly in the annulus [2]. This abnormal calcification of the valvular apparatus can lead to additional abnormal mechanical stress on the valve cusps further accelerating the valvular degeneration. The aortic valves usually are trileaflet with severe senile calcified degeneration. Although both the aortic valvular calcification and mitral annular calcification may result in significant valvular stenosis, clinically it tends to be more hemodynamically important with the aortic valve. The other interesting clinical finding is the occurrence of infective endocarditis. Most valves are structurally normal other than the abnormal calcification. However, in several series the indication for surgery is infective endocarditis in up to 20% of the cases, which is higher than in a nonrenal failure population. One explanation for this increase is related to the ongoing need for percutaneous access for dialysis therapy. Due to the continuous exposure to transcutaneous access there is always the possibility that these patients may develop transient bacteremia, which then seeds the heavily calcified valves with abnormal flow patterns. These factors—abnormal calcium and phosphate metabolism, hypertension, increased stress on valve leaflets, and possible intermittent bacteremia—may explain the association between the number of years on dialysis and the premature development of valvular heart disease in patients with ESRD.

Valve selection: mechanical versus tissue

For patients requiring valve replacement the selection of the type of valve prosthesis still remains somewhat controversial. The conventional wisdom for many years was that bioprosthetic valves would rapidly calcify and deteriorate requiring a repeat operation. This appears to be based on several reports from the late 1970s of calcification of porcine valves implanted in four dialysis patients [8,9]. Subsequently, mechanical valves became the valve of choice by many cardiothoracic surgeons [10–12]. However, over time and based on a larger although still limited clinical experience, this conventional wisdom has been reevaluated.

As the disease process associated with chronic renal failure was better understood, it became apparent that the 5-year survival was frequently limited in this patient population. Three of the most common causes of death in patients with ESRD are coronary artery disease, sepsis, and bleeding complications. In a review of Medicare patients with ESRD in the United States from 1982 to 1987, Byrne reported an overall survival of only 52% at 3 years and 33% at 5 years for patients between 55 and 65 years of age [13]. Based on such a limited overall survival, the issue of valve choice was slowly reevaluated. If many patients were not going to live beyond 5 years, was it really necessary to use a mechanical valve designed for longer use and requiring daily anticoagulation with warfarin therapy? Subsequently, many single-center reports comparing predominantly overall survival between bioprosthetic and mechanical valve replacement in patients with ESRD were published [14–17]. The general conclusion of all these publications was that there was no survival advantage with mechanical valves and frequently more complications related to the required anticoagulation. Although individually these reports still represented a relatively small experience, the growing consensus was that bioprosthetic valves were not contraindicated and should be considered for patients with ESRD who require valve replacement. At about the same time, Herzog and colleagues retrospectively reviewed the U.S. Renal Data System database to evaluate the current recommendation that a mechanical valve was preferred over a bioprosthetic valve in patients with ESRD [18]. In this report, there were 5858 dialysis patients who had valve replacement surgery. As expected, the majority of patients had mechanical valves and 881 patients had tissue valves. The conclusion from this study was once again that there was no difference in survival after cardiac valve replacement with tissue versus mechanical valves. Herzog and colleagues even went further and in their conclusions recommended that the current practice guidelines should be changed. In 2004 the Canadian Cardiovascular Society Consensus on Surgical Management of Valvular Heart Disease recommended bioprostheses for valvular replacement surgery in this patient population [19]. And just recently, the ACC/AHA guidelines have been changed to reflect the more recent clinical experiences and data suggesting that a bioprosthesis would be the favored choice in patients with ESRD [20].

It would seem then that the debate over the choice of valve, mechanical versus tissue, had been put to rest. However, there are still some conflicting reports, and the fact that most published reports are actually limited by the relatively small number of patients who were evaluated leaves some room for concern. For instance, in Jamieson's experience there was actually a statistically significant survival advantage in favor of mechanical prostheses at 5 years, yet the conclusion was that bioprostheses should be considered in these patients [16]. Also, the experiences from Japan are very different from the U.S. experience. Although there are differences in patient populations, Held *et al.* found that after adjusting for age and diabetes the relative mortality risk for ESRD in the United States was 15% higher than in Europe and 33% higher than in Japan [21]. The implication being that in Europe and Japan there may be many patients with ESRD that might outlive a bioprosthetic valve. Thus, there is still some concern about the general recommendation that a bioprosthesis is the valve of choice for any patient requiring valve replacement surgery with ESRD. Some have advocated a more individualized approach to choosing between a tissue and mechanical valve based on associated risk factors and that individual patient's expected long-term survival [22].

Aortic valve replacement

The etiology of aortic valve disease is most commonly from severe calcific degeneration as previously described. Therefore the majority of patients have aortic stenosis as the underlying pathology of the aortic valve. However, aortic insufficiency may be seen since endocarditis is the surgical indication for approximately 20% of patients requiring aortic valve replacement [14,15,17]. Coronary artery disease is frequently present and may require concomitant coronary revascularization. This is important as those patients requiring coronary revascularization in addition to aortic valve replacement have a decreased long-term survival compared to those patients having aortic valve replacement only.

Evaluating the morbidity and mortality of aortic valve replacement is complicated by the fact that most centers report on different time intervals and frequently give an aggregate mortality of valvular replacement with ESRD. Thus many reports on mortality are actually a combination of patients with either aortic, mitral, or double valve replacement surgeries. Table 1 demonstrates the difficulty in making general conclusions about the overall outcome for replacement of the aortic valve. As can be seen,

Table 1 Aortic valve replacement.

				Survival (%)		
Author	Yr	Pts	Op Mort	1 yr	3 yr	5 yr
Lucke	1997	12	16%	60		42
Smedira	2000	27	0%		36*	27*
					50[†]	33[†]
Craver	2002	55	3%[‡]	61	29	16[§]
Jamieson	2006	40	29%[¶]		22*	52[†]

*Survival for patients with bioprosthetic valves.
[†]Survival for patients with mechanical valves.
[‡]Although the operative mortality was reported as 3% the 3 month mortality was 27%.
[§]The 16% survival was at 6 years.
[¶]The early mortality was less for patients receiving mechanical valves (13.6% vs 36.2%) with an overall early mortality of 29%.

not all authors report on the mortality at the same time intervals and have relatively small experiences other than Herzog's review of the U.S. Renal Data System database. The overall cumulative experiences would suggest that there is significant 30-day mortality ranging from 0–29% and poor 5-year survival ranging from 20–50%.

Mitral valve replacement

Although many patients with ESRD develop severe calcification of the mitral annulus, it is even less common that it will require surgical repair than the calcified aortic valve. Experience with mitral valve replacement is subsequently very limited in busy, experienced heart surgery centers. As a representative example, in series published by Lucke, Smedira, Jamieson, and Craver [14–17] (Table 2), they have a total of 55 mitral valves that have been replaced. Once again, these mitral valve cases have not been evaluated as isolated procedures but have been grouped together with aortic valve replacements based on whether they received a tissue or mechanical prosthesis. Subsequently, the mortality that is reported is heavily weighted toward those patients who actually had the aortic valve replaced. As is true with mitral valve repair or replacement in a nonrenal failure population, the morbidity and mortality are not the same as for aortic valve replacement. Thus, it is reasonable to conclude that overall, isolated mitral valve replacement is relatively uncommon, the mortality appears to be similar to that for aortic valve replacement, and a tissue valve is worth considering given the poor short-term outlook. In addition, many of the patients may require coumadin anyway due to underlying atrial fibrillation, dilated left atrium, poor ventricular function, or ongoing access issues requiring anticoagulation for patency.

Table 2 Mitral valve replacement.

Author	Yr	Pts	Op Mort	1-yr survival
Lucke	1997	5	*	†
Smedira	2000	11	*	†
Craver	2002	30	*	†
Jamieson	2006	22	*	†

*Operative mortality was reported for combined group of aortic, mitral, and aortic/mitral valve replacement. No separate operative mortality was reported for isolated mitral valve replacement.
†No individual survival was reported for mitral valve replacement. Only aggregate survival was reported.

Mitral valve repair has been attempted in the past but with mixed results [23–25]. Due to the usually severe mitral annular calcification, it is difficult to perform an adequate annuloplasty. In addition, the degenerative calcific process is ongoing even after the repair, which further reduces the long-term success. Currently, there are few patients with chronic renal failure who would be candidates for mitral valve repair and the limited results are inconclusive.

Aortic and mitral valve replacement

Patients requiring both aortic and mitral valve replacement are even less common. The patients receiving both an aortic and mitral valve surgical replacement are probably selected with some bias since the morbidity and mortality for an isolated valve replacement are high. Despite the fact that most patients on chronic renal replacement therapy develop severe calcification of both the aortic and mitral valves, there are very few reported cases. Once again, using the series reported by Lucke, Smedira, Jamieson, and Craver, they have a cumulative total of 24 patients having both valves replaced [14–17]. The morbidity and mortality for the double valve replacements are grouped together with the isolated aortic or mitral valve patients making it difficult to determine a risk for these patients. As noted, these patients were probably selected as potentially low-risk patients since they did not seem to significantly affect the overall mortality in these selected series. In Herzog's review of the U.S. Renal Data System database, there were 562 (10%) combined aortic and mitral valve replacements over 20 years [18]. This would represent about 28 double valve replacements procedures per year on a national basis. Based on these estimates, it is safe to say that many cardiac surgery programs may rarely, if ever, perform this procedure. Although there are little data on the outcomes of these patients, the current recommendation that bioprosthetic valves have similar outcomes to mechanical valves and should be considered is applicable here as well.

Discussion

Renal failure requiring dialysis is an independent risk factor for any patient requiring valve replacement surgery [26]. Patients with chronic renal failure develop calcification of the aortic and mitral valves as part of the ongoing metabolic abnormalities associated with renal replacement therapy. It is more common that the calcification of the aortic valve apparatus will be hemodynamically significant compared to the mitral valve. Currently, most of the recently published information on the surgical outcomes for aortic or mitral valve replacements would indicate that bioprosthetic valves should be considered as the valve of choice based on the limited long-term survival of the group with fewer anticoagulation-related complications. However, it should be noted that there may be some patients who would outlive a bioprosthetic valve, may require warfarin therapy for other medical conditions, or may be a possible renal transplant patient in whom a mechanical valve may be preferred.

Most cardiac surgery programs currently have a limited experience with this high-risk group of patients requiring valve surgery. In addition to renal failure as an adverse risk factor, dyspnea at rest, dialysis for more than 60 months, combined procedures (CABG) and NYHA Class IV symptoms are found to be associated with a higher perioperative risk for death [27]. Since the majority of these cases are not emergent, it may be worth considering transferring these patients to busier cardiac surgery centers. This would allow the patients to have the best possible outcome and allow the accumulation of data from experienced centers so that future treatment decisions could be determined from evidence-based medicine rather than from isolated anecdotal experiences.

References

1 Pastam S, Bailey J. Dialysis therapy. *N Engl J Med* 1998;**338**(20):1428–1437.

2 Maher ER, Young G, Smyth-Walsh B, Pugh S, Curtis JR. Aortic and mitral valve calcification in patients with end-stage renal disease. *Lancet* 1987;**2**(8564):875–877.

3 Fulkerson PK, Beaver BM, Auseon JC, Graber HL. Calcification of the mitral annulus. *Am J Med* 1979;**66**(6):967–977.

4 Forman MB, Virmani R, Robertson RM, Stone WJ. Mitral annular calcification in chronic renal failure. *Chest* 1984;**85**(3):367–371.

5 Hammer WJ, Roberts WC, deLeon AC. "Mitral stenosis" secondary to combined "massive" mitral annular calcific deposits and small, hypertrophied left ventricles. *Am J Med* 1978;**64**(3):371–376.

6 Nestco PF, Depace NL, Kotler MN, *et al*. Calcium phosphorus metabolism in patients with and without mitral annular calcium. *Am J Cardiol* 1983;**51**:497–500.

7 Maher ER, Pazianas M, Curtis JR. Calcific aortic stenosis: a complication of chronic uraemia. *Nephron* 1987;**47**(2):119–122.

8 Lamberti JJ, Wainer BH, Fisher KA, *et al*. Calcific stenosis of the porcine heterograft. *Ann Thorac Surg* 1979;**28**:28–32.

9 Fishbein MC, Gissen SA, Collins JJ, Jr, *et al*. Pathologic findings after cardiac valve replacement with glutaraldehyde-fixed porcine valves. *Am J Cardiol* 1977;**40**:331–337.

10 Ko W, Kreiger KH, Isom OW. Cardiopulmonary bypass procedures in dialysis patients. *Ann Thorac Surg* 1993;**55**:677–684.

11 Zamora JL, Burdine JT, Karlberg H, Shenaq SM, Noon CP. Cardiac surgery in patients with end-stage renal disease. *Ann Thorac Surg* 1986;**42**:113–117.

12 Kaul TK, Fields BL, Reddy MA, Kahn DR. Cardiac operations in patients with end-stage renal disease. *Ann Thorac Surg* 1994;**57**:691–696.

13 Byrne C, Vernon P, Cohen JJ. Effect of age and diagnosis on survival of older patients beginning chronic dialysis. *JAMA* 1994;**271**(1):34–36.

14 Brinkman WT, Williams WH, Guyton RA, Jones EL, Craver JM. Valve replacement in patients on chronic renal dialysis: implications for valve prosthesis selection. *Ann Thorac Surg* 2002;**74**:37–42.

15 Kaplon RJ, Cosgrove DM, III, Gillinov AM, Lytle BW, Blackstone EH, Smedira NG. Cardiac valve replacement in patients on dialysis: influence of prosthesis on survival. *Ann Thorac Surg* 2000;**70**:438–441.

16 Chan V, Jamieson RE, Fleisher AG, Denmark D, Chan F, Germann E. Valve replacement surgery in end-stage renal failure: mechanical prostheses versus bioprostheses. *Ann Thorac Surg* 2006;**81**:857–862.

17 Lucke JC, Samy RN, Atkins BZ, *et al*. Results of valve replacement with mechanical and biological prostheses in chronic renal dialysis patients. *Ann Thorac Surg* 1997;**64**:129–133.

18 Herzog CA, Ma JZ, Collins AJ. Long-term survival of dialysis patients in the United States with prosthetic heart valves. *Circulation* 2002;**105**:1336–1341.

19 Jamieson WRE, Cartier PC, Burwash IG, *et al*. Canadian Cardiovascular Society. Surgical management of valvular heart disease. *Can J Cardiol* 2004;**20E**;1–120.

20 ACC/AHA 2006 guidelines for the management of patients with valvular heart disease: a report of the American College of Cardiology/American Heart Association Task Force on Practice Guidelines (writing Committee to Revise the 1998 guidelines for the management of patients with valvular heart disease) developed in collaboration with the Society of Cardiovascular Anesthesiologists endorsed by the Society for Cardiovascular Angiography and Interventions and the Society of Thoracic Surgeons. *J Am Coll Cardiol* 2006;**48**(3):1–148. (No abstract available; PMID: 16875962 [PubMed—indexed for MEDLINE]).

21 Held PJ, Brunner F, Odaka M, Garcia JR, Port FK, Gaylin DS. Five-year survival for end-stage renal disease patients in the United States, Europe, and Japan. *Am J Kidney Dis* 1990;**15**:457.

22 Ryuji HI, Yasmo TA. Cardiac valve replacement in patients on dialysis [letter to the editor]. *Ann Thorac Surg* 2002;**73**:696–697.

23 Chang JP, Kao CH. Mitral valve repair in uremic congestive cardiomyopathy. *Ann Thorac Surg* 2003;**76**:694–697.

24 Sim EKW, Mestres CA, Lee CN, Adebo O. Mitral valve repair in patients on chronic hemodialysis. *Ann Thorac Surg* 1992;**53**:341–342.

25 Lewandowski TJ, Armstrong WF, Bolling SF, Bach DS. Calcification and degeneration following mitral valve reconstruction in patients requiring chronic dialysis. *J Heart Valve Dis* 2000;**9**:364–369.

26 Edwards FR, Peterson ER, Coombs LA, *et al*. Prediction of operative mortality after valve replacement surgery. *J Am Coll Cardiol* 2001;**37**:885–892.

27 Horst MI, Mehlhorn UW, Hoerstrup SI, Suedkamp MI, de Vivie ER. Cardiac surgery in patients with end-stage renal disease: 10-year experience. *Ann Thorac Surg* 2000;**69**:96–101.

CHAPTER 6

Surgical evaluation and treatment of uremic pericarditis

Rosemary F. Kelly, Sara J. Shumway

Introduction

Uremic pericarditis is a known complication of end-stage renal disease. Although the etiology remains poorly understood, pericarditis in acute and chronic renal failure can present a significant hemodynamic risk with resultant morbidity and mortality. Chronic, intensive dialysis often results in resolution of this serious complication. However, even in the absence of azotemia pericarditis can occur. Pericarditis associated with end-stage renal failure can be classified as uremic, dialysis related, and constrictive. Both medical and surgical therapeutic options have been developed to manage this difficult problem.

Incidence

Pericardial disease associated with renal failure is relatively common. There is a wide spectrum of severity of pericardial abnormalities. Chronic renal failure produces an acute pericarditis that can be effusive or noneffusive, with or without tamponade, and often complicated by pericardial hemorrhage. Dialysis-related pericarditis is a chronic, recurrent pericarditis that may become a constrictive pericarditis. Acute renal failure is also associated with pericarditis, but usually of less serious consequence.

Pericarditis associated with end-stage renal disease is dramatic in both the rapidity of appearance and severity of the complications it may produce. In the era before dialysis, pericarditis was observed in 35–50% of uremic patients with chronic renal failure and much less frequently in acute renal failure [1]. Currently, the incidence of pericarditis in uremic patients that occurs prior to instituting dialysis has decreased to less than

10% [2]. This has been due in part to earlier diagnosis of renal failure with prompt institution of dialysis. Asymptomatic pericardial effusion in uremic patients prior to the onset of dialysis therapy is as high as 36% [3]. The occurrence of pericarditis after the onset of dialysis has remained fairly stable at 10–20% [2,4,5]. Dialysis-related pericarditis can occur at any time after a patient is stabilized on dialysis therapy, but 40% of cases develop in the first 3 months [4,6,7].

Etiology

The precise pathogenesis of all varieties of uremic pericarditis remains uncertain. No consistent biochemical differences have been found between terminally uremic patients with and without pericarditis [7]. However, multiple factors have been reported to contribute to the development of uremic pericarditis. The primary considerations include fluid overload, infection, and metabolic abnormalities of uremia [4,8]. In addition, metabolically stressful events such as trauma, infection, hypercatabolic states, or hyperparathyroidism may precipitate the onset of pericarditis [4,6]. The asymptomatic pericardial effusion in uremic patients appears related to volume overload [3]. This complication usually responds well to intensive dialysis. In glomerulonephritis, which may have an immunologic component for pericardial involvement, there is a clear association between the pericarditis and the cause of renal failure.

There are several confounding factors when trying to determine the etiology of uremic pericarditis. The diseases that cause renal failure, clinical conditions associated with renal failure, and medications used in the management of renal failure may all independently result in pericarditis and/or pericardial effusion. About 9.5% of episodes of pericardial effusion and pericarditis in uremic patients have been associated with systemic lupus erythematosus, Wegener's granulomatosis, rheumatoid spondylitis, and the use of minoxidil [2]. In addition, it is important to consider in the differential diagnosis myocardial infarction and ascending aortic dissection when evaluating a renal failure patient with a new effusion because these patients often have complicated medical situations. Other factors considered causative in uremic pericarditis include calcium [4], uric acid [9], and immune complexes [10]. Unfortunately, the evidence to support these possibilities is limited and inconclusive. It will require further investigation to define a clear etiology of uremic pericarditis.

Pericarditis that occurs once hemodialysis has begun and remained stable appears to be a unique entity. It can appear despite successful dialysis with appropriate fluid and biochemical correction of uremia. By definition, it occurs 2 weeks or longer after appropriate dialysis therapy has begun. Dialysis-related pericarditis occurs less frequently when peritoneal dialysis is used compared to hemodialysis. Why this is true may be related to the inflammatory state precipitated by hemodialysis. Circulating imine complexes, which may be pathogenic, are increased in hemodialysis patients especially those with various forms of serositis [11]. These imine complexes are less elevated with peritoneal dialysis. On the other hand, there are several considerations that support the concept of inadequate dialysis as a cause of dialysis-associated pericarditis. This is supported by the observation that increasing the frequency of dialysis leads to resolution of pericarditis in 50–70% of patients [2,4,7]. However, the fact that almost half of patients with dialysis-related pericarditis fail to have resolution despite increased frequency of dialysis suggests a more complex etiology [7,8]. An observation made at the University of Oklahoma was that the annual incidence of dialysis-related pericarditis increased in parallel with the incidence of influenza. The change in clinical management to include influenza vaccinations has resulted in a dramatic decline in the occurrence of pericarditis [12].

Development of pericardial effusion in association with the pericarditis occurs when fluid production from the inflamed pericardium exceeds reabsorption. This may be due to fluid overload associated with the renal failure or inflammation due to infection or inflammatory disease. Uremic exudates tend to have abundant amounts of fibrin and inflammatory cells. The fluid may be serous, hemorrhagic, or purulent. Pericardial contents are usually sterile unless secondarily infected. In uremia, there is abundant vascular granulation tissue accompanying the pericarditis as well as systemic hematologic impairments that promote bleeding. For this reason, the increased size of the pericardial effusion in uremic patients can somewhat predict increased risk of tamponade because the unstable uremic hemorrhagic diathesis can precipitate tamponade suddenly [13].

Presentation

The pericarditis of uremia or associated with dialysis has a typical presentation. Nonexertional chest pain is the most common presenting complaint and can occur in 76–100% of patients [2,14]. It is occasionally pleuritic with an increase in pain with recumbency and improves with sitting upright. Other symptoms of dyspnea, malaise, and cough are less frequently noted unless effusion or constriction is associated with the pericarditis. Pericardial effusion can occur without pericarditis; if it is noncompressing, it is usually asymptomatic.

Although the symptoms of pain due to pericarditis can precede objective evidence of pericarditis by 1–2 weeks, a pericardial friction rub is usually heard on examination at some point in the clinical course of uremic pericarditis. Fever occurs in less than 30% of patients [2]. Other signs are related to the presence of an associated effusion or constrictive pericarditis. These signs include increased jugular venous pressure and hypotension, often occurring at the time of dialysis. The increased jugular venous pressure occurs in the absence of tricuspid regurgitation. A characteristic feature is pulsus paradoxus. However, the pulse is not truly paradoxic, but rather demonstrates an exaggeration of the normal inspiratory decline in systemic blood pressure and pulse pressure. Although these signs are noted in patients with a hemodynamically significant effusion, neither is a reliable indication of cardiac tamponade. The speed of development of cardiac tamponade is highly variable. The vascular granulation tissue accompanying uremic pericardial inflammation is prone to bleeding given the uremia-associated hematologic impairments. This can precipitate sudden tamponade. Cardiac tamponade is a medical emergency, as the increased intrapericardial pressure limits ventricular filling and stroke volume, and thereby curtails an adequate cardiac output, despite compensatory tachycardia [15]. Death due to pericarditis in association with end-stage renal disease is related primarily to the development of pericardial effusion and resultant cardiac tamponade.

Noninvasive diagnosis of pericarditis and pericardial effusion

The diagnosis of uremic pericarditis, with or without effusion, is often made using only clinical history and physical examination. In the event of clinical suspicion without examination evidence of fever or friction rub, other diagnostic studies are necessary. The electrocardiogram may assist in establishing the diagnosis. However, the best study for making a definitive diagnosis is the echocardiogram.

There are classic electrocardiographic changes associated with pericarditis [15]. These changes are ST elevation in all leads except aVL and V_2, depressed aVR and V, and PR segments deviated opposite to P-wave polarity. However in uremic pericarditis, electrocardiograms often remain unchanged [2,13]. The typical electrocardiogram findings of pericarditis reflect subepicardial myocarditis, which is absent in uremia. This may be due to the fact that inflammatory cells do not penetrate the myocardium in uremic pericarditis. Indeed any "typical pericarditis" changes suggest positive viral pericarditis. Despite the lack of definitive changes in uremic pericarditis, the electrocardiogram is a critical diagnostic tool for chest pain in that it may reflect changes due to cardiac disease or metabolic abnormalities, both of which frequently occur in end-stage renal disease.

In regard to a pericardial effusion, the most common electrocardiogram finding is low voltage of QRS. Whereas low voltage in the electrocardiogram is common with pericardial effusion, the presence of effusion does not reliably alter the QRS voltage of the QRS complex. Interestingly, if electrical alternans is present with the effusion, it will disappear as the fluid is removed. Because of the limited ability to diagnose or quantify an effusion by electrocardiogram, echocardiogram is required for further evaluation.

Echocardiogram examination is the important diagnostic study in the evaluation of pericarditis. The echocardiographic changes of pericarditis are quite distinctive. There is increased echogenicity of the pericardium, which reflects a thickening of the pericardium. Pericardial thickness greater than 6 mm is diagnostic for pericarditis. In addition, the echocardiogram will demonstrate the presence of an associated pericardial effusion (>50 cm^3) in 90% of patients at some point during the clinical course of uremic pericarditis [2]. In the patient with a large effusion, cardiac tamponade is suggested by diastolic collapse of the right atrium and/or right ventricle. Echo-Doppler evidence of markedly decreased neutral and aortic valve flow velocities on inspiration further suggests impending cardiac tamponade [16].

The value of echocardiography is not only its diagnostic capabilities, but also that it is a highly reproducible and reliable means of defining and following effusive or constrictive pericarditis over time. Neither physical examination nor echocardiography provides totally reliable evidence of pericardial tamponade. However, by integrating the echocardiography findings with those of the clinical presentation it is possible to establish with reasonable certainty if tamponade or hemodynamic compromise is present. It is an important means of determining the effectiveness of dialysis therapy. Further studies such as chest computer tomography or cardiac catheterization are rarely indicated. Figure 1 demonstrates typical chest x-ray and echo findings of a large pericardial effusion.

Medical treatment

Since the introduction of dialysis management of end-stage renal disease, the incidence of uremic pericarditis has declined to 20% [8]. Initial management in the hemodynamically stable patient consists of intensive, daily hemodialysis [3]. A careful assessment of intravascular volume is critical as rapid vascular volume reduction in the presence of a large effusion

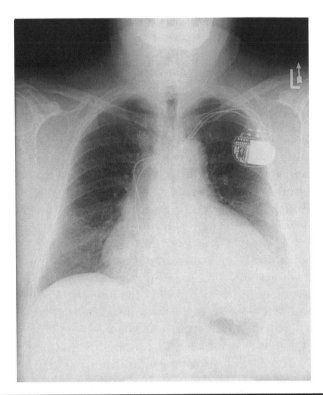

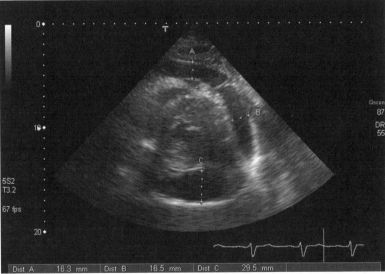

Figure 1 Chest radiograph and echocardiogram of a chronic dialysis patient who developed worsening shortness of breath over a one month period. The chest radiograph demonstrates an enlarged cardiac silouette without evidence of pleural effusion or pulmonary disease. Transthoracic echocardiogram confirms a thickened pericardium and a large pericardial effusion with evidence of stranding and loculation of the fluid. Percutaneous catheter placement may result in incomplete drainage of the effusion given the presence of loculations.

can precipitate cardiac tamponade. Intensive hemodialysis will be effective in approximately 70–80% of patients [2,17]. Patients who are prone to fail medical management include those with hypotension, elevated white blood cell count to greater than 15,000/mm [3], jugular venous distension, large effusion, or anterior as well as posterior effusion on echography [17]. Systemic corticosteroids have provided inconsistent, often only temporary, relief [4]. Indomethacin was found to be ineffective in a controlled double-blinded study [18]. Intrapericardial hydrocortisone, triamcinolone or an equivalent nonabsorbable agent may accelerate improvement by suppressing inflammation [19].

The algorithm for medical management of uremic pericarditis assumes that the patient is hemodynamically stable. If there is no associated effusion, or only a small effusion present, the patient is started on daily, intense hemodialysis. Monitoring by echocardiogram is critical to quantify the response to therapy. Usually an echocardiogram every third day will be adequate. If there is no resolution of a large effusion or an increase in the effusion size by 10–14 days of this management, then surgical intervention should be considered [2,8,17].

The development of new or recurrent pericarditis while undergoing chronic hemodialysis occurs in 10–15% of patients [2]. The initial management is again, intensive, daily hemodialysis as long as the patient remains hemodynamically stable. This therapy alone is 50–60% effective in complete resolution of pericarditis [2,4,7,17]. Again, a response to intense, daily hemodialysis is expected within 10–14 days [8]. Other therapeutic options such as changing to peritoneal dialysis, systemic steroidal therapy, or nonsteroidal anti-inflammatory agents may be employed, but each has limited and unproven efficacy. In those patients who fail to respond, there may also be evidence of progressively increasing pericardial effusions; sustained large effusions increased central venous pressure, development of rhythm disturbances, and development of incipient tamponade. Echocardiography assists in determining the response of the effusion to intensive hemodialysis. Careful monitoring by serial echocardiogram is essential in assessing the need for invasive intervention.

Pericardiocentesis can be a critical intermediate step in the management of uremic effusive pericarditis, particularly when there is evidence of impending cardiac tamponade. However, it should not be performed routinely. It is a conservative, though invasive, technique indicated for diagnosis of a purulent effusion or treatment of impending tamponade. The initial success in reducing the size of the effusion and in relieving hemodynamic compromise is around 80% [20]. The difficulty with pericardiocentesis alone is that recurrence occurs in the majority of patients. The instillation of steroids into the pericardium has been shown to improve long-term resolution of pericarditis with a decreased incidence of recurrent effusion [8]. Subxiphoid insertion of a needle into the pericardium, typically guided by electrocardiographic or echocardiographic control, enables removal of fluid and relief of the hemodynamic abnormalities of tamponade. Removal of even a small amount of fluid can produce striking hemodynamic improvement. Usually a small catheter is inserted via the needle into the pericardium for continued drainage. This assures a more complete drainage and provides a means of monitoring in the event of inadvertent injury to the heart.

The role of pericardiocentesis is controversial as there is significant risk associated with it in this particular patient population. The fibrinous nature of the exudate and frequent loculations may precipitate complications. In addition, the granulation tissue and bleeding diathesis associated with uremia make needle drainage of the effusion a higher risk procedure compared to pericardiocentesis for other etiologies. Finally, the difficulty of complete drainage due to posterior fluid collections or loculated collections can contribute to therapeutic failure. The major complications of pericardiocentesis occur during tapping and are caused by needle contact with the heart. Injury to the coronary veins, right atrium, or right ventricle is especially dangerous because the structures are thin walled and likely to bleed briskly producing significant hemopericardium. In rare instances, injury to the stomach, colon, and lung have occurred [13,21]. Also, as patients are vasotonic, a neurogenic reflex may contribute to postdrainage collapse. For this reason, atropine should be available at the time of the pericardial effusion drainage. These concerns make needle drainage of uremic effusive pericarditis a less attractive option. In the emergent situation of impending tamponade, the placement of a drainage catheter is recommended. This catheter also provides access for steroid instillation if desired.

Surgical management

Despite intensive medical therapy, uremic pericarditis may still progress to life-threatening hemodynamic compromise due to effusive or constrictive pericarditis. As noted, the results of pericardiocentesis can be temporary and associated with significant morbidity. Though effective, intense dialysis reduces the need for surgical intervention in this disease process, it is still an important component of management for select patients. When despite intensive dialysis, echocardiography demonstrates evidence of an enlarging or persistent effusion impending tamponade or recurrence of effusion after pericardiocentesis, surgical intervention is warranted. The optimal surgical approach and the degree of pericardial resection necessary remain controversial.

Surgical drainage and pericardiectomy can be accomplished by antero-lateral thoracotomy, median sternotomy, or video-assisted thoracoscopic surgery (VATS) [22,23]. Pericardiotomy via the subxiphoid approach allows for effective drainage of the pericardial effusion, but less access for lysis of adhesions. Surgical drainage of the pericardium is shown to be very successful in the long term for this problem as it has a greater than 90% effectiveness in resolving the constrictive or effusive pericarditis with a less than 3% incidence of recurrence [5,12,23].

Open thoracotomy approach for pericardiectomy has the advantage of removing the entire effusion as well as a sizable amount of pericardium to prevent late constriction. It also allows lysis of any adhesions. Access is through an anterolateral incision or median sternotomy. Both approaches yield excellent long-term results [12,14]. If there is the possibility of requiring cardiopulmonary bypass to complete the pericardiectomy safely, the technique of choice for constrictive pericarditis is median sternotomy. As uremic pericarditis is rarely associated with a calcified pericardium, this approach is rarely required. However, some surgeons prefer this approach due to the ease of complete pericardiectomy and lysis of adhesions [22]. However, the open procedures are associated with higher complication rates of pneumonia and cardiac arrhythmias [21]. The use of video-assisted thoracoscopic technology has reproduced the anterolateral approach, but there is limited reported experience and it seems appropriate only for effusive pericarditis [23]. With a VATS resection, a large portion of the pericardium and lysis of pericardial adhesions is possible. In addition, VATS has the advantage of smaller incisions with more limited postoperative pain. A well-established technique is the subxiphoid extrapleural drainage, which is highly effective and associated with low morbidity. It is a simple method of drainage in effusive pericarditis with low risk of recurrent effusion or developing late constrictive pericarditis [21]. It is an inappropriate approach for constrictive pericarditis as the exposure is too limited. Overall, surgical intervention in uremic effusive or constrictive pericarditis is an essential therapeutic intervention for patients who have failed medical management.

Summary

Uremic pericarditis continues to be a serious complication of end-stage renal disease. It can be an effusive or constrictive pericarditis. Fortunately, there is a decreased frequency of patients presenting with uremic pericarditis due to earlier diagnosis of renal failure with timely institution of dialysis. The incidence of pericarditis in patients on chronic dialysis has remained constant however. Medical management, which primarily includes increased frequency of dialysis, can often effectively treat this problem and is the first line of therapy. In our institution, surgical intervention for uremic pericarditis has become a fairly uncommon procedure. This reflects the importance of an early and aggressive dialysis regimen in the treatment of renal failure. Echocardiography is a critical study in this situation as it is the most accurate method to diagnose tamponade, progression of disease, or resolution in response to therapy. If the patient does not respond to medical management, further intervention is indicated. The role of pericardiocentesis is limited due to the difficulty with complete drainage and the associated risks of the procedure. Pericardiectomy remains the definitive therapy for effusive or constrictive uremic pericarditis that is unresponsive to medical management. It can be performed as an open procedure or by VATS. A pericardiostomy, via a subxiphoid approach, for effusive pericarditis can be equally effective.

References

1 Wacker N, Merrill JP. Uremic pericarditis and chronic renal failure. *JAMA* 1954;**156**:764–765.
2 Rutsky EA, Rostand SG. Pericarditis in end-stage renal disease: clinical characteristics and management. *Semin Dial* 1989;**2**:25–30.
3 Frommer JP, Young JB, Ayus JC. Asymptomatic pericardial effusion in uremic patients: effects of long-term dialysis. *Nephron* 1985;**39**:296–301.
4 Compty CM, Cohen SL, Shapiro FL. Pericarditis in chronic uremia and its sequels. *Am Intern Med* 1971;**75**:173–183.
5 Connors JP, Kleiger RE, Shaw RC, *et al.* The indications for pericardiectomy in the uremic pericardial effusion. *Surgery* 1976;**80**:689–694.
6 Baily GL, Hampers CL, Haber EB, *et al.* Uremic pericarditis: clinical features and management. *Circulation* 1968;**38**:582–591.
7 Marini PV, Hull AR. Uremic pericarditis: a review of incidence and management. *Kidney Int* 1975;**7**(suppl. 2):163–166.
8 Renfrew R, Buselmeier TJ, Kjellstrand CM. Pericarditis and renal failure. *Annu Rev Med* 1980;**31**:345.
9 Clarkson BA, Uric acid related to uremic symptoms. *Proc Eur Dial Transplant Assoc* 1966;**3**:3–8.
10 Twardowski ZJ, Alpert MA, Gupta RC, *et al.* Circulating immune complexes: possible toxins responsible for serositis (pericarditis, pleuritis and peritonitis) in renal failure. *Nephron* 1983;**35**:190–195.
11 Maisch B, Kochsiek K. Humoral immune reactions in uremic pericarditis. *Am J Nephrol* 1983;**3**:264–271.

12 Frame JR, Lucas SK, Pederson JA, *et al.* Surgical treatment of pericarditis in the dialysis patient. *Am J Surg* 1983;**146**:800–803.

13 Gunukula SR, Spodck DH. Pericardial disease in renal patients. *Semin Nephrol* 2001;**21**:52–56.

14 Robertson JM, Mulder DG. Pericardiectomy: a changing scene. *Am J Surg* 1984;**148**:86–92.

15 Shabetai R, Fowler NO, Guntheroth WG. The hemodynamics of cardiac tamponade and constrictive paricarditis. *Am J Cardiol* 1970;**26**:480.

16 Appleton CP, Hatle LK, Popp RL. Cardiac tamponade and pericardial effusion: Respiratory variation in transvalvular flow velocities studied by Doppler echocardiography. *J Am Coll Cardiol* 1988;**11**:1020–1030.

17 De Pace NL, Nestico PF, Schwartz AB, *et al.* Predicting success of intensive dialysis in the treatment of uremic pericarditis. *Am J Med* 1984;**76**:38–46.

18 Spector D, Alfred H, Siedlecki M, *et al.* A controlled study of the effect of indomethacin in uremic pericarditis. *Kidney Int* 1983;**24**:663–669.

19 Buselmeier TJ, Davin TD, Simmons RL, *et al.* Treatment of intractable uremic pericardial effusion: avoidance of pericardectomy with local steroid instillation. *JAMA* 1978;**240**:1358–1360.

20 Morin JE, Hollomby D, Gonda A, *et al.* Management on uremic pericarditis: a report of eleven patients with cardiac tamponade and a review of the literature. *Ann Thorac Surg* 1976;**22**:588–592.

21 Rostand SG, Rutsky EA. Pericarditis in end-stage renal disease. *Cardiol Clin* 1990;**8**:701–707.

22 Arsan S, Mercan S, Sariqul A, *et al.* Long-term experience with pericardiectomy: analysis of 105 consecutive patients. *Thorac Cardiovasc Surg* 1994;**42**:340–344.

23 Nakamoto H, Suzuki T, Sugahara S, *et al.* Successful use of thoracoscopic pericardiectomy in elderly patients with massive pericardial effusion caused by uremic pericarditis. *Am J Kidney Dis* 2001;**37**:1294–1298.

Index